"Dr. Joel Fuhrman is a rising star in the medical community. His program for vibrant health and his approach to healing should be integral parts of every physician's standard prescription. A diet of fruits, vegetables, grains, and legumes allows the body's own rejuvenative powers to work, often with surprising results. And fasting has shown a remarkable effect in conditions that may have been thought to be virtually untreatable. Dr. Fuhrman's powerful and practical guidelines apply for conditions ranging from the common cold to serious heart problems. This program provides an alternative to the cost and all-too-common side effects of surgery and drugs."

—ANDREW NICHOLSON, M.D.,
Director of Preventive Medicine
Physicians Committee for Responsible Medicine

"By individually tailoring nutrition plans based on a case-by-case basis, Fuhrman has treated hundreds of patients with rheumatoid arthritis successfully."

—*Vegetarian Times*

"As a family physician who has used nutrition and healthy lifestyle as the basis of my practice for over ten years, I believe that the information in Dr. Fuhrman's book is essential for every practicing physician who genuinely wants to get his sick patients well and keep his well patients from getting sick. Although some physicians give lip service to the value of health promotion, the profession as a whole has little idea of the tremendous degree to which lifestyle affects health and disease. The result is that people are unnecessarily sick, and expensive, high-tech treatments are not making them well. Dr. Fuhrman presents a better solution in this book. *This is where the future of medicine should be heading*."

—RONALD CRIDLAND, M.D.

D0182145

"Dr. Fuhrman's approach is a refreshing change from the high-tech, symptom-oriented, medical and surgical treatments that dominate medical care today. This is neither alternative medicine nor conservative medicine, but rather progressive medicine. By aiming his treatment at the underlying causes of many chronic diseases rampant in our society, Dr. Fuhrman's approach offers individuals suffering from these diseases the only real chance for a meaningful cure. I have been fortunate to observe many of these outcomes firsthand and can testify to the power of this approach for certain diseases."

—JAMES CRANER, M.D., M.P.H.

"Dr. Fuhrman's book is revolutionary. It shows clearly and un-mistakably the way to recover health, and could change the prevailing way of treating disease."

—THEODORE COUMENTAKIS, M.D.

"If you are lucky, you will read Dr. Fuhrman's book before you have subjected yourself to medications and medical procedures. This book is for those who want to take charge over their health and well-being, for those who want to embark on a journey towards a more satisfying life."

—DAN JERET, M.D.

"As a family physician who deals with chronically ill people on a daily basis, I know that every health seeker in America will want to read this book. It provides a working knowledge of vital information that is currently known to relatively few people. Share it with those you love."

—JOHN PILLA, M.D.

"Finally, a modern-day, scientific book about fasting and nutritional intervention to reverse disease. It will be nothing less than a complete revolution in health care, watching millions throw away their medication and get well when the information in this book is utilized by our society. Every person in America must learn about this safe, non-invasive approach for getting well. Nothing else can equal the ability of the therapeutic fast to unleash the healing potential within every patient."

—GEORGE FETT, M.D.

"Dr. Fuhrman's book places the ancient healing practices of diet and fasting into the hands of modern practitioners—and their patients. Thought-provoking and sure to be controversial, this guide will be seen as one of the mileposts on our journey towards sane, affordable health care, based upon simpler and more natural methods. It will be valued by anyone seeking more vitality, a greater understanding of their body, or aid in overcoming a personal health challenge."

—MICHAEL KLAPER, M.D.

FASTING
—AND EATING—
FOR HEALTH

A Medical Doctor's Program for Conquering Disease

JOEL FUHRMAN, M.D.

St. Martin's Griffin ❧ *New York*

Note to the reader
The information provided in this book is intended to describe the potential benefits of a natural diet and therapeutic fasting. However, any decision involving the treatment of an illness should be made only after consulting the physician of your choice. Do not start, stop, or change medications without professional medical advice, and do not change your diet if you are ill or on medication, except while under the care of a physician. Neither this nor any other book should be used as a substitute for professional medical care or treatment.

Fasting—and Eating—for Health is not meant to be a how-to guide to self-conducted fasting. Readers should take important note that all fasts should be conducted under the supervision of a qualified doctor trained in the use of therapeutic fasting.

The names of patients discussed in this book have been changed, along with certain identifying characteristics.

Design by Janet Tingey

Library of Congress Cataloging-in-Publication Data

Fuhrman, Joel.
    Fasting and eating for health : a medical doctor's program for conquering disease / Joel Fuhrman.
        p.   cm.
    ISBN 0-312-18719-X
    1. Fasting—Therapeutic use.   2. Diet therapy.   I. Title.
RM226.F84 1995
615.8′54—dc20
                                                    95-12430
                                                        CIP

10   9   8   7   6   5   4

I dedicate this book to Lisa, my wife of thirteen years. Her support and encouragement have enabled me to pursue my personal visions and helped make this book a reality. Without her devotion to our three beautiful daughters, I would not have had the peace of mind to devote myself to the project of writing this book, on top of the sixty hours a week I spend in my medical practice.

Acknowledgments

This book would not have been possible without earlier work by pioneers of nutritional healing, especially Herbert Shelton.

I greatly appreciated the help in editing this book from my sister, Elen Weiss. My friend Max Huberman also spent many hours editing and offering sage advice. I am sincerely in debt for his gracious help.

Doris Walfield also made valuable contributions to the manuscript.

I will always be grateful to my father, Seymour Fuhrman, who, more than anyone else, influenced my thinking about health. His conviction and enthusiasm for learning about health science spurred my interest.

I thank my three daughters, Talia, Jenna, and Cara, for their cooperation in allowing me to write this book. They have graciously sat by my side or on my lap while I worked at the computer.

Contents

Foreword

A revolution is occurring in the world of modern medicine. We now have powerful tools against conditions that previously had defied our strongest medical treatments. Where drugs and surgery have failed, these emerging techniques bring results that surprise the doctor and delight the patient.

Joel Fuhrman, M.D., is leading that revolution. He is one of the most remarkable physicians in America, and it is no surprise that many doctors, including me, often refer patients to him and call on his advice. Dr. Fuhrman is not only an expert in modern medical diagnosis and treatment, but also has developed a unique expertise in strengthening the body's innate abilities to restore health, often from very serious conditions, without the need for medications. Dr. Fuhrman is putting these techniques within the reach of everyone.

We all know that our bodies naturally rebound from a cold or "flu." Our white blood cells seek out and destroy the invading viruses, and all we have to do is get out of their way and let them work. But our ability to restore good health goes much further than that. Built into our cells are natural mechanisms that can clean cholesterol, fat, and debris from our arteries; restore health to joints that are attacked by arthritis; and bring us to a level of health that we may never have anticipated. The key to unleashing these wonderful functions lies in the nutrients the body has to work with.

As Dr. Fuhrman shows us, the right nutrients can turn on these abilities, while the wrong nutrients—which are all too common in the standard western diet—can leave these abilities buried forever. The most amazing results, however, come when the body is given a complete rest from the work of digestion and assimilation of food.

Therapeutic fasting goes back thousands of years, of course, and was long regarded by doctors as being more appropriate for philosophers than physicians. Researchers, however, have investigated what occurs when the body takes a short break from nutrients. They have studied the biochemical events that occur in the bloodstream, in the joints, in the fat tissues, and in the brain, and have found astonishing results.

Rheumatic arthritis, for example, has long challenged physicians. Existing drugs are too weak to change the course of the disease, and are usually used to make the patient more comfortable as the joint destruction progresses. But several teams of researchers have shown that within days of beginning a supervised fast, the joints cool down, and as the foods that triggered the arthritis are identified and then avoided, the disease often disappears, never to return.

Scientific journals have now embraced this knowledge, and a growing number of doctors are putting it to use in their daily practice. Individuals should work with these doctors, rather than fast on their own, because while fasting is safe, it is also powerful and should be monitored as health returns.

Dr. Fuhrman is foremost in this new generation of medical leaders. The information he provides in this volume is clear and practical and of vital interest to patients and doctors alike.

I am grateful to Dr. Fuhrman for assembling this remarkable work, and recommend it to you wholeheartedly.

NEAL D. BARNARD, M.D.
President, Physicians Committee for
Responsible Medicine

Fasting
—and Eating—
for Health

Introduction

Therapeutic fasting accelerates the healing process and allows the body to recover from serious disease in a dramatically short period of time. In my practice I have seen fasting eliminate lupus and arthritis, remove chronic skin conditions such as psoriasis and eczema, heal the digestive tract in patients with ulcerative colitis and Crohn's disease, and quickly eliminate cardiovascular diseases such as high blood pressure and angina. In these cases the recoveries were permanent: fasting enabled longtime disease sufferers to unchain themselves from their multiple toxic drugs and even eliminate the need for surgery, which was recommended to some of them as their only solution.

As a means for recovery from disease, fasting has hit the front pages of major medical publications due to its recognized effectiveness in well-controlled scientific studies. Although fasting has been around as a therapeutic approach for thousands of years, only now is the medical profession studying the broad-reaching reparative properties of the fast. Even with this progress, most of the medical community and the general public are still unaware that the medically supervised fast is the safest and most effective treatment for many dangerous but common illnesses.

The health of our nation is not improving; in fact, we are getting sicker. Changes are developing in health care, and the public is more aware that a problem exists. Our economy is weighed down by an expensive and largely ineffective medical system that relies on expensive tests, treatments, and last-minute heroics to attempt to combat the harmful effects of a nation poisoning itself with a rich, disease-causing diet.

The U.S. Public Health Services, in a progress report of its "Healthy People 2000" program to reduce the prevalence of chronic disease in the nation, found no improvement in the overall dietary practices of Americans between 1976 to 1980 and 1992. This conclusion is based on data from the National Health and Nutrition Examination Survey and the U.S. Department of Agriculture. In fact, we now have the most overweight population in the history of mankind. Medical propaganda to the contrary, our adult population has never been sicker, and cancer rates have continued to climb.

While high-tech methods such as new drugs and surgical techniques (angioplasty and bypass surgery, for example) aim to reduce symptoms, they do not address the underlying cause of the disease, and people are getting sicker and sicker. The underlying cause I am referring to is not an absence of adequate medical care. It is severe malnutrition. By malnutrition, I do not mean the lack of food or nutrient deficiency; rather, what we have today is a society of overfed people, poisoning themselves with high-fat, high-protein, highly refined foods. This rich diet harms our bodies and lays the groundwork for chronic degenerative disease. Fasting in conjunction with optimal nutrition after and before the fast offers the ability to undo the damage done to the body by the rich diets of modern societies.

In the last ten years there has been a revolution in medicine. The diet–disease relationship is more well documented than ever before. More and more physicians are embracing nutritional and preventive approaches. Doctors are advising their patients about the quality of their diets and about the importance of exercise and life-style modifications such as smoking cessation. The physician community and the population are attempting to modify cardiac risk factors by lowering their intake of fats and cholesterol. Even dietary suggestions for reducing the risks of cancer are in vogue.

New information, collected from large investigations on various human populations, has shown that the majority of the chronic and life-threatening diseases are preventable. But because conventional medical therapy does not address the cause of disease, it thereby limits itself greatly as a long-term solution.

Because of conventional medicine's limited success and high costs, alternative treatments are becoming more widely used. Fasting, combined with nutritional competence, removes the most significant causes of disease and, due to its great success, is now being looked at by conventional physicians as well as by patients. The health care of the future will have to be both more effective and less costly than what we have available today. Fasting, as a therapeutic modality, is safe, effective, and a true health care bargain.

In most serious chronic diseases the body can heal itself and recover when a properly conducted fast is undertaken. Certainly there are advanced pathologic states, such as cancer, that will not respond to fasting, but the majority of chronic diseases do respond in a predictable manner. Modern medicine offers little hope of recovery from the variety of chronic debilitating diseases affecting the population. Fasting offers that hope.

Many current approaches offered by the medical profession to deal with a medical problem or health crisis involve significant risk or side effects. Fasting is noninvasive and can be both more effective and safer than the more standard approach. The details of this with regard to multiple disease states will be explained in this book. Additionally, the traditional medical practice of treating the symptoms of a disease with medicine or surgery does not remove the causes. Inevitably these causes, left unchecked, allow the disease process to advance. By contrast, therapeutic fasting, supported by a healthy life-style, removes the causes of disease and accelerates the healing process. This can allow the disease sufferer to reclaim a normal life, free of a lifetime of medicines and further suffering.

As you read this book you will experience the thrill of learning all about the miraculous healing powers of the human organism.

The self-healing power of the body is often overlooked because it is rarely given a chance to act in a world that expects the quick fix. The power of the body is as evident as green grass, rainy days, and sunshine. It is by no means a mystical power: it arises from the same exceptional intelligence that produced you out of two microscopic cells and that heals your wounds when you are injured. It is the same set of natural human characteristics that allows you to eliminate waste or to "lose weight" when you change your diet. It is the same innate ability that allows an exhausted individual to go to bed (without eating) and wake up vibrant and full of energy for another 16 hours. Fasting enables the body to repair and rejuvenate its own tissues, by directly providing the conditions for recovery and removing the impediments that curtail your recuperative powers. The fast establishes a unique opportunity, vital for the restoration of health.

I will present many case histories in this book in order to give you factual knowledge about how fasting can help get you healthy . . . fast. After reading these pages you will be clear on how to act efficiently in putting your life on the fast track of healthy living.

I present this case history now as an illustration of why I am so enthusiastic about fasting and why I feel it is so vitally important to share this information with everyone.

Years ago, a 20-year-old world-class athlete and Olympic ice skating hopeful suffered a severe injury to his leg. Forced to walk on crutches, he could not bear weight on his leg without excruciating pain. His heel was so swollen and sensitive that the mere weight of a bed sheet caused intense discomfort. Because he was ranked among the top two in the country in his event, the U. S. Olympic Committee encouraged him to seek treatment by one of the country's leading orthopedic surgeons.

After months of prodding, probing, and medical tests by the prominent doctor, and still unable to walk after a year in pain, the young man was quite discouraged. His doctors offered him no solution to the swelling and acute sensitivity in his injured foot. Then one day without warning, while in the hospital, a nurse instructed him to take a medication because the doctor intended to perform surgery the following morning. Outraged, the young man refused to take the drug and demanded that his physician discuss the proposed surgical plans with him.

Later that day, the doctor stormed into the room and brusquely informed the athlete that experimental surgery was required to promote the healing of his foot. The doctor explained that after exposing the injured tissues, he would use his scalpel to traumatize the area in a checkerboard pattern in an attempt to stimulate the area to heal. When the young man refused to participate in such an experiment, the physician angrily told him that if he did not have the surgery he would never walk again. Nevertheless, the young man rejected the surgery and left the hospital.

The young athlete was aware that a few years earlier his arthritic father had restored his health by fasting. He remembered the articles and books he had read on fasting at that time and realized that the technique probably offered his best chance to recover.

Determined to give fasting its best chance, he traveled to Dr. Shelton's Health School in San Antonio and fasted a total of 46 days. At the end of the fast he was able to walk again. In a little over a year he placed third in the World Professional Figure Skating Championships.

At Dr. Shelton's Health School, the young man saw asthmatics cured so they no longer needed medication. He met colitis patients with bleeding bowels who recovered without drugs or surgery. He observed people with chest pain who had been told they needed bypass surgery. They were riding bicycles and jogging for the first time in years. The young man saw for himself how the body could heal itself if the causes of disease were removed.

This man was so impressed with what he witnessed and experienced that he sought out other practitioners who used fasting and natural diets to heal patients. What he learned from them excited him so much that he later decided to attend medical school and become a physician. At medical school, however, the patients were treated with conventional modern methods. Given large amounts of medication to control their symptoms, they rarely got well. No cardiac patients stopped taking drugs because their angina disappeared. No hypertensive patients stopped taking medication because their condition improved. No arthritic patients recovered and threw away their pills.

As a medical student, the young man saw patients suffer and die needlessly, while under the care of modern medicine. Through it all, he remained convinced that people could get well if only they knew how to use fasting and natural diet to restore their health.

This young man was I.

1 | **Fasting for Physical Rejuvenation**

Many thousands of people have restored their health through therapeutic fasting. Some, ill and distraught from years of discomfort and discouragement, try fasting as a last resort. Fortunately, the majority of people who undergo a supervised fast not only improve or recover (often from what are considered incurable diseases) but also experience physical, psychological, and mental rejuvenation. Fasting to heal oneself can mean the difference between living life pain-ridden and dependent on drugs, going from one doctor to another for relief, and living a normal pain-free existence into old age.

Therapeutic fasting is not a mystical or magical cure. It works because the body has within it the capacity to heal when the obstacles to healing are removed. Health is the normal state. Most chronic disease is the inevitable consequence of living a life-style that places disease-causing stressors on the human organism. Fasting gives the body an interlude without those stressors so that it can speedily repair or accomplish healing that could not otherwise occur in the feeding state.

Fasting stops the continual work of the digestive tract, whose activity can drain the body of energy and divert the healing processes. Each time we take in food, the body must secrete digestive enzymes to break down the food, move these simpler components into the cells lining the digestive tract, and further move these nutrients into the bloodstream for distribution throughout the body. All of these functions require a substantial amount of vitality and energy—energy that might otherwise be used to fuel the healing process.

Each time we take in food we take in not only nutrients but also additives and other toxins. The digestive tract, the liver, the kidney, and other organs must work to remove these non-nutritive substances from the body. These wastes include by-products of digestion, bacterial by-products from the decomposition of inadequately digested foodstuffs, and excess nutrients the body cannot use. All these as well as the waste products of normal cellular metabolism must be actively eliminated for us to maintain excellent health.

Food, therefore, while providing essential nutrients for life, also introduces toxins. Fasting, particularly when we are ill and the body is already overburdened with self-produced wastes, can provide a welcome relief by halting the introduction of further toxins and waste products. Without this extra burden, the body is finally able to heal itself.

Individuals who suffer from chronic disease often have weakened or abnormal digestive function. Indeed, this is often the reason they are ill to begin with. In these cases, fasting allows the digestive tract to take a much needed break to restore itself to normalcy.

When a person's appetite and hunger disappear, especially during an acute illness, the loss of appetite indicates that the body has a much lowered capacity for digestion. Forcing this person to eat can result in the absorption of partially or improperly digested food, which will impede a quick and complete recovery.

What Is Fasting?

Fasting, in the strictest sense, is defined as the voluntary abstinence from all food and drink, except water, as long as the nutritional reserves of the body are adequate to sustain normal function. This is a state of relative physiologic rest. Some of the medical studies on fasting (which we will refer to) have included the use of vitamins, coffee, tea, and drugs during the fast. Except for extremely rare instances where some medication may be indicated, it should be recognized that a total fast, with water only, is both the most effective and the safest way to fast.

Vitamins are not generally required because within the body's cells are adequate reserves of protein, fat, minerals, and vitamins that can be called upon during periods of famine, food scarcity, or fasting. Even in prolonged fasts (those lasting from 20 to 40 days) no deficiency diseases develop, illustrating that the body has the innate ability to utilize its stored reserves in a highly exacting and balanced manner. Today, with modern laboratory tests available, it is simple to check the blood for levels of every vitamin and mineral, as well as for electrolytes and other essential factors. Interestingly, these levels of vitamins and minerals are exceedingly stable during the fast and, if normal to begin with, remain normal throughout the period of fasting.

In some cases a liquid diet, such as fruit or vegetable juices, has been considered to be a fast. This may occasionally be appropriate for a person who requires relative bowel rest, whose health condition would make a fast inappropriate. One cannot, however, achieve the powerful benefits of complete fasting if juices are part of the fast. "Juice fasting" is not truly fasting; biochemically the body does not enter the "protein-sparing" fasting state. In this state the body conserves its muscle reserves and fat is preferentially broken down. This does not occur with juice fasting. Juice fasting also does not have the powerful anti-inflammatory properties of the pure water fast that are essential for recovery in autoimmune illnesses. Other benefits of total fasting include decreasing platelet aggregation and promoting other biochemical changes that help to prevent the formation of blood clots, which could cause a heart attack. These beneficial changes, so essential in the cardiac patient, as well as the significant lowering of blood pressure, also do not occur if even a small amount of carbohydrate in the form of juice is taken.

Occasionally claims are made for special powders, vitamin preparations, herbal mixes, or drinks that are intended to detoxify the liver more effectively than fasting. Obviously, this is wishful thinking. The powerful detoxifying effects of the fast cannot be obtained by following a restricted or supplemented diet. Only when there is total abstinence from all calories do we observe waste products being heavily excreted from the breath, the tongue, the urine, and the skin. Plus, the fast does not merely detoxify, it also breaks down superfluous tissue—fat, abnormal cells, atheromatous plaque, and tumors—and releases diseased tissues and their cellular products into the circulation for elimination. This kind of dramatic detoxification cannot occur with supplemented eating plans. Toxic or unwanted materials circulate in our bloodstream and lymphatic tissues and are deposited in and released from our fat stores and other tissues. An important element of detoxification is mobilizing the toxins from their storage sites. This occurs best and most efficiently during total fasting.

I have observed many sick patients who have tried these "detoxification" powders and not achieved results. I have seen how easily these same people recover when they go on a complete fast. We can't buy magic in a bottle. A supplemented powdered drink food plan may sometimes be helpful for a person with food sensitivity or a very poor diet, but I find that in these cases, where total fasting is not necessary, changing the diet alone almost always achieves equally good results, and adding supplemental nutrients is practically never needed.

To think that we can buy an herb that will detoxify us is also an illusion. Herbs do not detoxify. They merely are a source of nutrients or natural drugs. For example, they do not detoxify the liver or kidney when they increase urinary output. *Diuretic* is the name given to a drug that can increase our urine flow. When a drug functions as a diuretic it does so because of its ability to block or poison the ability of the cells that line the kidney's collecting ducts to reclaim fluid. When a natural herbal diuretic is taken, it works via the same mechanism. Instead of accurately referring to it as a diuretic, its proponents call it a kidney strengthener or detoxicant. Obviously, the profit motive encourages claims made for many so-called "healing" substances. It is attractive to think we can buy good health in a bottle, but unfortunately it is not that easy. There is nothing that can be taken that will ever accomplish the biochemical changes that occur when we undergo a complete fast.

Nature Has Designed the Human System with the Capacity to Fast

The human body has been designed to fast safely. Certain biochemical changes take place when no food is taken that enable the body to fuel itself by burning up its fat reserves and conserving its vital tissues. As this book illustrates, the design of the human system is so masterful that it has built into it the blueprint to change its fuel consumption to fast safely.

The innate intelligence of the body is remarkable, as represented by the biochemical changes that occur in the fasting state. Glucose is a simple sugar that supplies the necessary fuel our body needs. Normally, if we don't eat for a day or two, we start to utilize muscle tissue to make the glucose needed by the body, since glucose can be manufactured from amino acids stored in our muscles. If we continue to fast, however, the body senses what is occurring and attempts to conserve its lean muscle mass by a few different mechanisms.

Fats are broken down to fatty acids that can then be utilized by the muscles, heart, and liver for energy. The brain, however, is the major utilizer of energy when the body is at rest. The brain cannot be fueled from fatty acids; it requires glucose to fuel its operations.

A special adaptation occurs in the fasting state whereby the brain can fuel itself with **ketones** instead of glucose. By the third day of a total fast, the liver starts generating a large quantity of ketones from the body's fat stores. As the level of ketones rises in the bloodstream, the brain and other organs begin to use these ketones as their major fuel, thus greatly diminishing the utilization of glucose by the body. This significantly limits muscle wasting. These keto acids are utilized for fuel primarily by the brain, muscle tissue, and the heart.

This production of ketones, called ketosis, develops within 48 hours in females and 72 hours in males, and muscle wasting at this time decreases to very low levels. This is known as **protein sparing.**

Thus, the human organism responds to the fasting state by attempting to maximally conserve its muscle and lean body tissue. With severely restrictive diets, like juice fasts, the body does lose weight, but the brain and other organs do not subsist mainly on ketones. Therefore, proportionately to weight lost, juice fasts and severely restrictive diets cause us to lose more lean body tissue and less fatty tissue than do total fasts.

What Is Starvation?

Contrary to what many people believe, fasting is not starvation. **Starvation** begins when abstinence is continued beyond the time when the body's stored reserves are used up or have dropped to a dangerously low level. During the fasting stage the body supports itself from the stored reserves within its tissues. When food is eaten at normal intervals, the body stores sufficient amounts of nutritive matter to last for a rather lengthy time during later periods of abstinence. Even thin people carry a reserve of nutrients in their tissues to tide them safely over a period of fasting.

The body will not starve or in general even be hungry while fasting because it is "eating." It is consuming the substances the individual consumed last week, last month, and last year that have been converted into body tissue. In fact, the *symptoms* of hunger generally disappear by the second day of the fast. This illustrates that the body has entered a fasting, and (lean) tissue-sparing metabolism. Of course, there is a limit to the body's reserves. When they have been used up, specific symptoms occur that indicate the fast should not be continued.

The time required for a fast to reach completion varies from individual to individual. The trained physician can easily denote symptoms that indicate the ending of the fasting period and the beginning of starvation. In the vast majority of fasts, the physician will end the fast many weeks before the nutrient reserves of the body have been exhausted. The average individual (not over-weight) would have to fast approximately 40 days or more to exhaust nutrient reserves.

Such a prolonged fast is almost never recommended and, there-fore, we are not remotely considering the biologic processes of starvation during the fast of average length. If the fast was con-tinued beyond the point when the body's nutrient reserves were exhausted, starvation would begin. If not eating was continued past this point, damage to the body and even death could result. Most patients are fasted one to four weeks depending on their nutritive reserves and the purpose of the fast.

Fasting Is Nature's Restorer

In the animal kingdom, fasting is quite common. Some animals fast during hibernation or estivation (sleeping throughout the summer in tropical climates). Some animals fast during the mating season and in many cases immediately after birth and during the nursing period. Animals instinctively fast when sick or hurt. The ill or wounded animal finds a warm secluded spot where it can lie quiet and undisturbed to rest and fast for a period of time until health is restored. The ill animal sips only water until well again. Nature, with her superior wisdom, has provided the animal world with an instinct to do that which will facilitate optimal physical well-being.

Most people do just the opposite of the animals when they are sick. They maintain their hectic work schedule, continue to eat a rich diet, and take anything they can find to gain comfort. Any drug advertised to hide their signs and symptoms is ingested. Drugs, well recognized as toxic and harmful if ingested when we are well, are suddenly seen as healthful and healing when the body is suffering with an acute illness.

Many people are unaware that symptoms such as a runny nose or fever are the treatment the body has prescribed to remedy the condition. Increased mucus production is the body's means of washing away infected cells and removing virus particles from the body. Fever aids in the body's immune defenses, activating the white blood cells and inducing interferon secretion from the brain. Interferon is a powerful substance that stirs the fighting arm of the immune system into action. Typical cold symptoms that people attempt to suppress with drugs are nothing more than attempts of the body to restore homeostasis and remove the disease itself. By drugging away their symptoms, people keep themselves sick longer and can even turn a minor disease into a major one.

Rather, we should do as the animals do. We should listen to our bodies when appetite is diminished or absent. If we are not feeling well, we should sip water and rest. It is amazing how quickly patients recover from viral syndromes when this advice is taken. Recovery in this case leaves the body in a clean and healthy state, rather than contaminated with toxic medications; we have thus laid the groundwork for future good health.

In both acute illnesses and chronic disease there is no greater delusion than that an individual needs "strength" to fast. What is true is that such people have bodies that are too weak to digest the food they take in. The people who are most helped by a fast are those who are in most need. Too often the weak patient is told he or she must eat to regain health or strength. In many cases, while feeding, the person remains ill and fatigued.

Frequently, even extremely thin individuals who have been losing weight while feeding themselves rich foods show a tremendous improvement in their digestive capacity and begin to gain weight and strength after a moderate-length fast. Fasting enables them finally to reach a normal weight. This illustrates their weakened powers of digestion or assimilation or the presence of serious chronic disease such as digestive impairment or autoimmune illness, which improves or resolves as a result of the fast.

The job of fasting is to supply the body with the ideal environment to accomplish its work of healing. During the period of a fast the blood pressure will drop, the level of retained metabolic wastes will fall, and the blood vessels will begin to soften and rid themselves of hard sclerotic plaque. In a short period of time the heart and brain, as well as other organs and muscles, will receive a more adequate blood supply and oxygenation. The tissues throughout the body's systems will begin to purify themselves and the rejuvenation process of the fast will have begun.

The goal of the body at all times is to keep the individual healthy. When the disease-causing stresses are removed, the natural healing and self-repairing powers of the body begin to work unhindered. Within a short period of time, allergic and mucus-filled individuals clear their nasal passages, asthmatics breathe easier, arthritis sufferers report their pain is resolving, and cardiac patients begin to have increased circulation to their hearts. Healing has begun.

Healing and rejuvenation occur because fasting is an opportunity for the human body to take a rest from all of the stressful elements of life, such as physical labor and emotional stress. It is also an opportunity for the internal organs and digestive system to take a physiological vacation.

In our society, most people eat heavy foods during much of their waking hours. This not only overworks the digestive tract, but also forces the body to continue its work of digesting and absorbing foodstuffs and eliminating food-derived wastes well into the night. This prevents the body from totally directing its energies toward repair and self-cleansing of its tissues.

To regain normalcy or health, individuals suffering from chronic illnesses must rid their systems of the burdens of toxic material and excesses, such as fatty or swollen tissues or atherosclerotic plaque. It may be possible, over time, to eliminate the excesses while on a restricted diet that calls for taking in foods that support the body. Fasting, however, offers a much more efficient means of accomplishing healing that is dependent on the elimination of retained waste. This is because fasting gives the body an opportunity to focus completely on the elimination of the waste deposits and the purification of its tissues that are necessary to reach a recovered state of health.

When no calories are consumed, the body is living off its nutritional stores, primarily its fat reserves. The innate wisdom of the body is such that, while fasting, it will consume for its sustenance superfluous tissues, carefully conserving vital tissues and organs. The body's wondrous ability to autolyze (or self-digest) and destroy needless tissue such as fat, tumors, blood vessel plaque, and other nonessential and diseased tissues, while conserving essential tissues, gives the fast the ability to restore physiologic youth to the system. By removing or lessening the burden of diseased tissue, including the fatty tissue narrowing the blood vessels, fasting increases the blood flow and subsequent oxygenation and nutrient delivery to vital organs throughout the body.

Conceptually, fasting provides a comparative rest for the digestive tract, while, throughout the entire body, from the blood vessels and nerves in the feet to the noxious retained substances irritating the central nervous system, the body conducts an internal "spring cleaning." Fasting enables the entire system to focus on the elimination of superfluous tissue and the retained waste that it was unable to break down and remove in the feeding state.

When an individual has a serious chronic disease, we need to combine a fast with necessary dietary changes before and after the fast to achieve a recovery. By combining the fast with a healthy diet and life-style, the individual can maintain the benefits from the fast and remain healthy.

Fasting Is Not New

Fasting has been used as a healing modality throughout recorded history. Socrates, Plato, Pythagoras, and Hippocrates, for example, all recommended fasting for various physical conditions.

Our species has survived on the earth for the last 400,000 years partially because of the incomprehensible design of nature that enables us to survive under various circumstances, including going without food for prolonged periods of time. Built into our genetic code is the ability to instruct the body exactly what to do to survive in a period of famine, food scarcity, or natural disaster when food is unavailable for prolonged periods. Obviously, the body functions normally for quite a long time when no food but only water is ingested.

Extended religious fasts were frequently practiced by followers of far eastern religions and in the early days of Christianity, especially during the Middle Ages. Many of us have heard of individuals who have fasted for political reasons. Mahatma Gandhi, for example, fasted 21 days to promote Hindu–Moslem unity and mutual respect and tolerance between religions. Gandhi was actually very familiar with the scientific and health-related literature regarding fasting and even read the writings of and corresponded with Dr. Herbert Shelton, who conducted more than thirty thousand fasts on his patients earlier in this century.

Occasionally we hear of entombed miners, shipwrecked sailors, or stranded aviators who are forced to go without food for weeks and weeks. People survive for extended periods of time, until they are rescued, as long as they have access to nonsalt water.

So fasting is not new. It has been practiced for religious, political, and health reasons for thousands of years and has been recognized throughout recorded history as having a curative effect on sickness and disease. Mark Twain wrote in *My Debut As a Literary Person* (1889), "A little starvation can really do more for the average sick man than can the best of medicines and the best doctors. I do not mean a restricted diet: I mean total abstinence from food . . ."

For more than ten thousand years fasting has been utilized to heal the sick. Hippocrates regularly prescribed fasting for numerous conditions. The famous **Hippocratic Oath,** familiar to every physician, admonishes us to "First do no harm," recognizing that the most important foundation of healing the sick, even today, is the remarkable recuperative power inherent in the human body. This power of self-repair is beautifully witnessed during the fast.

Is Fasting Uncomfortable?

The reason many people are so afraid of fasting and find the mere thought of it so unpleasant is that when they skip even one meal they feel awful. They assume fasting would be very uncomfortable. These individuals—who exhibit uncomfortable signs early in the fast—are in greatest need of a fast. Headaches and other discomforts brought on by not eating are signs that the body has begun to withdraw from and detoxify waste products retained in body tissues. When we delay eating or fast, these tissue stores of toxic waste are mobilized for removal. Thus fasting is "cleansing" of the internal system. These detoxification symptoms usually do not occur in those who are in excellent health, with a lower level of retained wastes. When one is prepared properly with a low-fat, lowered-protein, natural, plant-centered diet prior to the fast, these symptoms, which actually are nothing more than withdrawal symptoms from a more rich diet, usually do not occur.

Fasting is not so uncomfortable as many would think. Hunger typically goes away completely by the second day and the symptoms of withdrawal from food and toxins typically end quickly, usually by the second day of the fast. Interestingly, it has been noted by physicians conducting fasts for decades that true hunger is a mouth and throat sensation, felt in the same spot that one feels thirst. Gnawing in the stomach, stomach cramping, headaches, and generalized weakness from not eating or skipping a meal or two are experienced only by those who have been eating the standard American diet with all its shortcomings (those most in need of a fast). Those who have been consuming a healthier, low-fat, low-protein, plant-based diet for months prior to the fast typically experience no such typical hunger pains when they fast.

Symptoms such as abdominal cramping and headaches, traditionally thought of as hunger symptoms, are not really symptoms of hunger. The medical books are obviously wrong here. These symptoms are experienced only by those eating a diet far too rich and stressful for their own internal controls. These symptoms are signs of withdrawal that indicate healing is beginning when the body has the opportunity to rest from the continual intake of food.

Detoxification and Improvement in Organ Function Occur Simultaneously

Nothing is more fascinating than watching toxins being rapidly discharged from the system while a person fasts. In fact, fasting has been employed to treat chemical poisoning by people who have recognized the powerful effect it has on accelerating the discharge of internal noxious wastes. One such enlightening use of fasting was the subject of an article in the *American Journal of Industrial Medicine* in 1984 entitled "A Trial of Fasting Cure for PCB Poisoned Patients of Taiwan." The study involved patients who had ingested rice oil contaminated with PCBs. After a seven- to ten-day fast, dramatic relief was noted and improvement in symptoms was reported by all patients.

Fasting also has a powerful effect on improving liver function. This benefit is not limited to the fasting period but continues after the fast. Medical studies have tested the ability of the therapeutic fast to improve conditions such as alcoholic liver injury, damage from fatty liver, and drug-induced liver injury. Dramatic improvements were consistently reported.[1]

Fasting is a very valuable treatment for psychological disorders. There are hundreds of journal articles in the medical literature documenting the value of fasting in improving the function of the entire body, including the brain[2,3,4,5]. Fasting has been repeatedly observed to alleviate neuroses, anxiety, and depression.[6] It appears from these studies that fasting improves our ability to adapt to frustration and external stress. One Japanese clinic fasted 382 patients with psychosomatic disease with a success rate of 87 percent.[7]

When the beneficial effects of the therapeutic fast were investigated with various research parameters measuring organ function, it was found repeatedly that substantial improvements are seen in the autonomic nervous system, endocrine system, and adrenal function after the fast.[8]

Fasting Typically Achieves Results Where Other Methods Have Failed

Many who earnestly want to improve their health are convinced that their diets are lacking in some vital nutrient or other substance that they can buy to recover their health. Though it may be true that some individuals, especially the elderly, may be borderline deficient in certain nutrients, the reality is that most of the chronic diseases people suffer from are not primarily the result of nutrient deficiencies. Therefore, supplying additional nutrients does not result in recovery. After a while, those with chronic medical conditions, including cardiovascular disease, migraines, colitis, arthritis, psoriasis, asthma, and sinusitis, realize that they still have not achieved a recovery and that they cannot purchase optimal health at the health food store or pharmacy.

The diets that I prescribe for my patients are abundant in appropriate nutrients, yet contain no excess of sugar, protein, fat, or cholesterol. Generally, by following an optimal diet and lifestyle, which will be described in the next chapter, chronically sick people get well. The rate of recovery from the diseases that have been mentioned, as well as from many other autoimmune and diet-related illnesses, is astonishing. While dietary modifications alone may be enough for recovery from disease in some cases, to obtain a complete recovery a physician-supervised fast often becomes the only solution to enable the individual to achieve the desired healing in a reasonable time frame. A properly conducted fast is a safe and expedient way to remove excesses from the body—excesses that are preventing the body from achieving a full recovery. Medications cannot do this.

Some persons who are suffering from serious chronic ailments can make great strides in their health while continuing to eat. It is important that these individuals strive to remove all the possible causes of ill health. This must include reducing all the stressors on the body, and calls for careful management of the diet (adapting it to their individual digestive and nutrient needs), less food, less work, and more rest. This method can frequently take too long and require infinite diligence and patience. A successful outcome is not so certain as when a prolonged fast is undertaken.

Sometimes people are not careful enough with the changes in their diet or are unwilling to make the changes that are sufficient to bring about a complete recovery from their condition. Then, when their health is restored with a fast and they see the health potential that is available to them through natural methods, they develop a heightened ability to conform to a healthy way of life to maintain their long-sought-after good health.

For those who are not in need of a fast, the very principles behind the fast are the basis for dietary changes that will lead to recovery and the subsequent control of health. Throughout this book the concepts of health recovery and disease causation that apply to both the fasting and the eating state will be explained. Readers will gain a clear comprehension of the causes of disease and how to maintain and achieve optimal health, even if they never fast.

The medical profession's primary method, over the last century, for combating the effects of improper diet and life-style has been to offer medication and surgery. This approach has not been effective. Almost every medical treatment offered for the chronic disease sufferer today attempts only to control symptoms. There are no "cures." The current medical treatments not only have risks, but also represent a Band-Aid type of approach—they can offer relief from symptoms but they cannot cure because they do not address the cause of the disease. Under "modern" medicine, the incidence of most chronic diseases has increased and the vast majority of people are still dying from what are preventable, diet- and life-style-induced illnesses.

Obviously, traditional medical treatments can be lifesaving in an emergency situation, and on some other occasions can be appropriate and extremely beneficial. We certainly have today the best emergency medical care ever available. But, overall, modern medicine has continued to fail. People are still suffering needlessly and dying prematurely. This is because treatments don't eliminate the primary cause: a rich diet that stresses the system and overloads the body with excesses and toxins.

Imagine if every day I smashed my hand with a hammer. Could I expect a pain medication or anti-inflammatory drug to heal the wound? Obviousy, I would not recover unless I stopped the daily pounding. Every day our nation's people are pounding themselves with a rich diet, ill-adapted to the needs of our species. This inevitably results in the eventual breakdown of our internal systems and the development of chronic disease.

Fasting, as opposed to the usual medical treatments, helps to remove the cause of the disease. For example, with atherosclerosis (the buildup of plaque in the arteries), fasting allows the body to work to actually remove the plaque from within the blood vessels. In diseases such as rheumatoid arthritis, fasting clears out the waste deposits that are stimulating the immune system and inflaming the joints. This allows the body to heal itself.

In addition to the consistently positive results of fasting on disease, fasting enables the disease sufferer to drop weight rapidly to a safer level. Excess weight in those suffering from diabetes, high blood pressure, high cholesterol levels, or angina can contribute to their premature death from a heart attack or stroke. While diets of every description flood the media, nothing will remove these risk factors more effectively, more quickly, or more predictably than fasting.

A natural foods dietary approach, utilizing superior nutrition, combined with therapeutic fasting, when appropriate, is the only way our society will be able to free itself from the hordes of ill people still chronically suffering and taking multiple drugs as the only option to lessen their symptoms.

The practice and methods described here offer a rational approach that is not only effective but also consistent with the Hippocratic admonition to "do no harm." The results described are consistent with natural laws and logic that would assume that health will result from healthful living and from removal of the causes of disease. Likewise, abuses done to our bodies, whether recognized or not, can result in ill health. Rather than merely reduce the signs of disease, such as lowering blood pressure with medication, this approach enables the faster to remove the disease itself and significantly extend longevity.

Doctors leave medical school with the hope and intent of gaining self-satisfaction through helping others in need. Doctors and patients both, however, become resigned and frustrated due to the inherent weaknesses in today's approach that calls for powerful diagnostic tests, and then leaves the patient with little option but to take potentially harmful drugs to attempt to control the signs and symptoms of disease. Rather than hoping for the discovery of some wonder drug, we are discovering the true wonder of the healing properties inherent in the human body that can be unleashed by removing impediments to normal function.

Once you are exposed to the powerful effects the methods described within this book will afford you, there is no turning back. As a result of reading this book, you will come to view your own body in a completely different way and will inevitably take better care of yourself in the future. The clear comprehension of the causes of disease and how to maintain and achieve optimal wellness will crystalize in your mind, giving you a powerful tool to regain control of your own health even if you never undergo a fast.

2

Improper Nutrition: The Major Cause of Disease

Man lives on one quarter of what he eats. On the other three quarters lives his doctor.

—INSCRIPTION
ON AN EGYPTIAN PYRAMID,
3800 B.C.

Modern research has confirmed the folk adage that eating less, and especially eating less fats and high-protein animal foods, prolongs life.

Our rich, modern diet has been implicated as a causative factor in cancer, heart attack, stroke, hardening of the arteries, and diabetes; and the leading causes of death in this country can be prevented or delayed by adopting healthier nutritional habits. The same foods that cause premature deaths also subject us to misery and chronic illness in life.

This is the main purpose of this book: to provide a more complete understanding of the cause of various diseases and to explain how to remove the obstacles to healing so you can recover your health.

If individuals choose to undergo a fast for internal cleansing and rejuvenation of their system, or for therapy of a specific disease, they must combine the fast with a healthy diet before and after fasting to maintain the benefits they reap from the fast. In many instances the change in diet alone is sufficient to achieve a complete recovery.

Many do not comprehend the relation between their food intake, their life-style habits, and their chronic illnesses, such as arthritis, osteoporosis, recurrent infections, allergies, acne, asthma, and sinusitis. Ironically, and sadly, health authorities, most physicians, and dieticians recommend the very same eating plans that cause these diseases to develop in the first place. Patients and their physicians generally rationalize that the problems they are facing are genetic, biochemical, structural, or otherwise beyond their control. Patients are frequently told the food they consume has nothing to do with the disease from which they suffer. This is simply untrue. Most chronic medical problems are not only caused by improper diet and life-style, but also can be *reversed* by adopting a more primitive and natural diet, one that our species was originally designed for.

This information is not a "new breakthrough" or medical discovery. Many renowned physicians, after reviewing the evidence collected over the last few decades, are taking a new approach to dietary recommendations. For example, the Physicians Committee for Responsible Medicine, headquartered in Washington, D.C., has recently asked the Department of Agriculture to replace the traditional four food groups (meat, dairy, grains, and fruits and vegetables) with four new ones: fruits, vegetables, grains, and legumes. The reasoning behind this change is sound—it emphasizes the foods that protect against disease rather than those that cause disease.

Unfortunately, we live in a modern society where suffering from preventable illnesses and chronic disease is the "norm." Half of us die from the totally avoidable occurrence of heart disease, and the majority of the individuals who do not die of hardening of the arteries die of cancer. Millions suffer from osteoporosis, deterioration of the musculoskeletal system, and chronic back and joint pain. The majority of people in this country are out of shape and overweight, and live their lives waiting for some disease to strike.

From hay fever and allergies to hypertension and high cholesterol, all these chronic conditions can be prevented through optimal nutrition. We do not need to be a nation of medical dependents, visiting physicians and taking drugs in a futile attempt to combat the effects of our disease-producing modern diet.

Instead of feeding ourselves in such a manner as to cause our deterioration, I recommend eating primarily unrefined plant foods. This means eliminating or de-emphasizing meat, chicken, fish, and dairy products; and avoiding processed foods, fried foods, fats, and sweets. If these rich foods are to be consumed at all, my patients are encouraged to limit their use to special occasions (once weekly or less) or to use animal-based foods only as condiments, in very small quantity, to flavor a soup or vegetable dish.

Even though these recommendations may be abhorrent to certain individuals and to the animal agriculture community, it cannot be denied that vegetarian populations live longer and healthier lives than meat-eating populations. Not only does the epidemiologic evidence from around the globe point to this, but also the studies on healthy vegetarian populations show that there is a significant survival advantage when animal foods are eliminated from the diet.[1,2]

Meat and dairy products, which have traditionally been our primary source of protein, have high fat and cholesterol content, minimal fiber, and are deficient in the cancer-preventing antioxidant nutrients. This nutritional profile of animal foods is the precise combination associated with an increased risk of coronary artery (heart) disease, most cancers, diabetes, and obesity.

Plant foods have substantial amounts of fiber, little fat, and moderate amounts of protein. Much modern research has linked not only fats to cancer and degenerative illnesses but also the proteins in animal products.[3] These foods were thought in the past to be appropriate for our species, but now it is clear that animal-based foods, because of their link to so many of our ills, are poorly adapted to humans when used in significant quantities.

As a species we are closely related to the great apes, who are primarily plant eaters. Clearly, the diet for which our species is best adapted is one consisting predominantly of natural, unrefined, plant-based foods with little if any foods of animal origin.

We're Winning the Race to an Early Death with Our Knives and Forks

Our population is nutritionally miseducated. Outdated nutritional concepts encourage us to feed our children a diet that promotes premature growth and rapid maturity. Nutritionists have suggested humans need to consume high-protein animal foods such as eggs, meat, and fowl because these foods have been noted to promote more rapid growth in rats and other rodents. This is a tremendous error, as now we have learned that growth acceleration promotes aging.

Over the years researchers noted that the rodents that matured and grew the quickest died the earliest. This was tested again and again with all animal species: the faster an animal grows and matures, the younger it dies.[4] This is now an established fact in humans as well; for example, early puberty increases our risk of certain cancers, especially breast and prostate cancer.[5]

It was also noted that if we restrict the calories an animal can eat, by underfeeding it or periodically fasting it, we can significantly prolong its life. In fact, periodically fasting animals can double their natural life span.[6,7]

Utilizing the traditional four food groups as a guide, modern society consumes a diet with a severe excess of fat, cholesterol, and protein, and that is also significantly deficient in fiber, vitamins, and minerals. Almost any menu that uses these outdated guidelines would have us consume between 30 and 45 percent of calories from fat. This is more than double the amount consumed in countries that do not have the high rates of heart attack and cancer that we see in our country today. Our fiber intake hovers around 10 to 20 grams per day, less than a fourth of what it should be.

The modern way of eating sets the stage for our bodies to function at low efficiency, stressing our internal organ systems, leading to chronic disease. Though all chronic diseases may have genetic factors contributing to their expression, without the stresses of modern living and modern dietary practices, these inherited differences, the weak links in our genetic codes, need never express themselves in chronic disease.

Chronic diseases, more prevalent in modern times, are on the rise not merely because people are eating an animal-based diet, but also because the grain products we consume are highly refined and processed to make them nearly devoid of fiber. In addition, modern societies consume a large amount of added sweeteners, simple sugars, and refined vegetable fats or oils. These foods rob us of our nutritional reserves and add further toxic stress to the body.

Rather than eat unprocessed foods as nature intended, most of us consume large quantities of processed foods that are high in fat, salt, sugar, and chemical additives and that are deficient in fiber and essential nutrients. Instead of providing a diet predominating in fresh fruits and vegetables, which supply the proper nutrients for normal development, most parents allow their children to consume large quantities of "empty-calorie" foods. These deficient foods include bottled fruit juice and other sweet drinks that are high in sugar and deficient in essential nutrients. Incredible as it may seem, the top three sources of calories in most American diets today are milk, cola, and margarine, with the combination of fat and refined sugar occupying 65 percent of caloric intake.[8]

It amazes me that the human body can even survive this onslaught of abuse that begins at such a young age. Is it any wonder that almost from birth many children are frequently sick with one infection after another? Then they get older, develop hay fever, allergies, or asthma, and are increasingly prey to autoimmune illnesses and cancer. Is it surprising that we have a nation of the walking sick? Unfortunately, few comprehend the correlation between diet and a multitude of common diseases such as acne, hyperactivity, anxiety, headaches, and PMS.

Obesity in children is also rising at an alarming rate. The May 1987 issue of the *American Journal of Diseases of Children* reported a 54 percent increase in obesity in 6- to 11-year-olds since 1960. The 1992 *Bogalusa Heart Study* discovered atherosclerotic lesions, the early signs of clogging of the arteries, in most children, teenagers, and young adults.[9] Autopsies were conducted on over 60 percent of all children who died, mostly by accidental deaths. They confirmed that this disease process begins very early in life, setting the stage for a premature death later on.

It astounds me that parents in our society allow their children to consume the foods they do—sugary cereals, fast food, pizza, white bread, and other empty-calorie foods, never wondering why their children are chronically ill, allergic, asthmatic, or have recurrent ear infections. High-calorie malnutrition takes its toll, flooding doctors' offices with sick patients of every description.

Pasta Is Not Health Food

The standard American diet is centered around animal foods and processed wheat products, neither of which are ideal foods. Even worse, the typical modern eater consumes a tremendous amount of extracted vegetable oil. Many Americans add high-fat dressings or sauces to almost everything they consume that is not a high-fat food to start with. Yet those familiar with the scientific research on fats, including extracted plant fats such as olive oil and soy oil, know that fats increase our risk of cancer.[10] Vegetable fats are processed foods that interfere with the normal function of our immune system[11,12] and that contribute to obesity and chronic disease.

When individuals change from an animal-food-based diet to a vegetarian diet, but then eat mostly processed foods such as low-fat pizza, tofu dogs and other health food store concoctions, refined cereals and grains, pasta, and bread as the primary source of their calories, the diet is still inadequate.

Grains, when consumed in their refined state, are comparatively poor sources of vitamins, especially antioxidants. They are also nearly devoid of essential fatty acids. The opposite can be said of green vegetables. Green vegetables and especially the leafy greens are rich in vitamins, minerals, and essential fatty acids, as well as thousands of other important nutrients that research scientists are beginning to identify as being essential for optimal health. These plant-based substances, called **phytochemicals,** support our immune system and protect us from cancer.

Just a few years ago, scientists didn't know phytochemicals existed. Today they represent the new frontier in cancer-prevention research. The reality is that there exist thousands of compounds that will never see the inside of a vitamin bottle. Until recently nobody even knew they existed, and more are being discovered each year. Every slice of an orange, every bit of broccoli, every forkful of romaine lettuce, contains thousands of these essential nutrients produced when sunlight hits plants. Only through eating large amounts of many different natural, unprocessed fruits and vegetables will we obtain these necessary elements for optimal health.

The normal functioning of the intestinal tract depends on the presence of adequate fiber. The typical diet is unhealthfully deficient in fiber. So another benefit of a diet high in natural plant food and complex carbohydrate is that it's invariably accompanied by more fiber. A diet high in fiber holds fluid within the digestive tract and moves feces through the system at a faster speed. This is important to protect against colon cancer, diverticulosis, appendicitis, and hemorrhoids, as well as constipation and intestinal spasm.

The contemporary diet that most Americans view as "healthy" is a far cry from that. Those believing they are on a "low-fat" diet are usually consuming between 30 and 40 percent of calories from fat, roughly three times as much fat as we should be eating. When the fiber and antioxidant nutrients consumed by most people are totaled, the result is frightfully low.

In a nationwide survey, only 9 percent of those polled had eaten three or more servings of vegetables and two or more servings of fruit on the previous day. People are not following the recommendations by the government to consume more fruits and vegetables. More important, even if they followed the U.S. Department of Agriculture's recommendations to the letter, their diet would still be inadequate. Though an improvement over the past, the recommendations of the new Food Guide Pyramid still do not sufficiently emphasize fresh fruits and raw and cooked vegetables.

The suggested guidelines still encourage a diet too high in fat and protein, and too low in plant-borne nutrients and fiber for optimal health. Only a plant-centered diet can provide optimal amounts of vitamins, minerals, and fiber while keeping fat intake under 20 percent of calories. For example, the diet I recommend supplies about 1,500 mg of vitamin C daily from food. With the abundance of fresh fruits and vegetables and the adequate amount of food-borne vitamin C come the other bioflavonoids and important unidentified compounds that are present only in whole plant food.

The Recommended Dietary Allowance (RDA) for vitamin C is 60 mg a day. This is a ridiculously low and arbitrary number, as are the RDA's of many other plant-derived nutrients. These inadequate recommendations are healthy only for the industrial food giants, so their products don't look as deficient as they are. Contrary to popular belief, we can get very large quantities of nutrients such as vitamin C, beta carotene, and vitamin E in our diets without the use of pills simply by eating a natural, plant-based diet.

Humans Were Not Designed to Eat Processed or High-Protein Foods

Our population has accepted the fact that more than half of us will die of heart attacks and more than a third will develop cancer at some point in our lives. So too is it accepted that we live and suffer with medical problems, take medications recommended by our physicians, and then die or become a physical or mental cripple in later years.

This common pattern is a tragedy of modern life, but one that can be avoided. Disease, dementia, and disability associated with aging are unnatural. We have control over our health as we extend our life span by making different food choices. Dennis Burkitt,

M.D., one of the world's most renowned physician researchers on human nutrition and a pioneer who established the value of fiber, has explained that western man has made more change in his diet over the last six or eight generations than has been made throughout the whole of the rest of his sojourn on earth.

Genetically, anatomically, and physiologically our bodies are the same as those of humans who lived in the Stone Age. What we put into our bodies is quite different. Refined supermarket food is being fed to our Stone Age bodies.

Much of the food found in supermarkets derives its calories from extracted sweeteners, sugars, fats, and refined flour. Besides the empty-calorie drawbacks and fat-producing effects of these foods, they are deficient in the vitamins, minerals, and other important nutrients needed by the body to burn them for energy. Therefore, the body must continually draw on its reserves of stored nutrients, thus draining its nutritional reservoir.

Not only sweets, but also all processed foods that no longer carry with them the essential nutrients endowed by nature are deficit inducing. For example, the ingestion of processed foods has been shown to induce chromium deficiencies, even though the chromium levels may have been normal before the introduction of these refined products.[13] Diets with a high ratio of refined carbohydrate to total carbohydrate induce various nutritional deficiencies. This form of high-calorie malnutrition causes the brain and nervous system to become irritable and the immune system to malfunction.[14,15] This weakens our immune system and has an assortment of negative effects on our development, including heightened intraocular pressure and poor eyesight.[16]

The **China-Oxford-Cornell Study** is one of the largest nutritional research projects ever conducted. This massive project, called the "Grand Prix of Epidemiology," documented the observation that in underdeveloped areas where populations consume predominantly unrefined plant foods, the degenerative diseases of modern society as well as the leading cancers are virtually nonexistent. This study confirms hundreds of other studies that have documented that most diseases of modern society originate from dietary folly. Unfortunately, the rural societies examined in the China-Oxford-Cornell Study are more and more adopting the "American way" of eating and are statistically beginning to show increasing incidence of disease.

The **China Project** dramatically demonstrates that if we plot the amount of animal foods eaten against the death rates from the leading causes of death (heart disease and cancers), all animal food consumption, even fish and chicken, raises the rates of cancer and heart disease.[17] Interestingly, even small quantities of animal foods in the diet were able to trigger higher cholesterol levels, heart disease, and cancer. The evidence from the **China Project** and other confirming studies shows that the animal protein itself, not just the fat in the animal foods, causes cholesterol to rise and cancer to increase. Dr. T. Colin Campbell, head of the **China Project,** predicts that in the next 10 to 15 years research will solidly establish that animal protein is one of the most toxic nutrients for humans.

Dr. Campbell has explained, "There is strong evidence in the scientific literature that when a reduction in fat is compared to a reduction in protein intake, the protein effect on blood cholesterol is more significant than the effect of saturated fat. Animal protein is a hypercholesterolemic agent . . . Many Americans are switching from beef to skinless chicken and other animal-based foods simply to reduce their intake of fat. However the existing evidence suggests that this makes little or no sense."[18]

It is clear that one should consume protein in quantities sufficient to meet the needs of the body, but with no extra. Excess protein affects the body in a variety of negative ways, shortening potential life span. Animal protein consumption has been linked with increased cancer rates and tumor formation as well as the acceleration of atherosclerosis.[19] Excess proteins also increase our requirements for other nutrients by reducing the uptake of folate, pantothenic acid, and pyridoxine, and by washing away essential minerals through the kidney as the kidney attempts to eliminate the extra nitrogenous waste.[20]

Because our physiological nature is such that we are primates, equipped with the virtually identical digestive apparatus (comparatively small liver and kidney) as the great apes, our structure is not well equipped to handle high quantities of concentrated fats and proteins. Monkeys also do poorly on high-protein diets and improve physically and emotionally when a high-carbohydrate diet is resumed.[21] Relatively high levels of uric acid, ammonia, and other toxins such as phenols, skatole, and indole are formed by proteolytic bacteria, which line our digestive tract when we consume a high-protein diet.[22,23] These toxic by-products elaborated by bacteria in our gut can significantly add to the toxic load the body must deal with on a daily basis and can contribute to multiple disease processes.

The idea that the major diseases in prosperous countries are related to dietary excesses is becoming a majority view among those studying the question. Dr. Mark Hegsted, Professor of Nutrition at the Harvard School of Public Health, stated before a Senate Committee, "The risks associated with eating this diet (rich in meat, other sources of fat, sugar, and refined carbohydrates) are demonstrably large. The question to be asked is not why should we change our diet, but why not? Ischemic heart disease, cancer, diabetes, and hypertension are the diseases that kill us. They are epidemic in our population. We cannot afford to temporize. We have an obligation to inform the public of the correct food choices. To do less is to avoid our responsibility."[24]

We continue to pretend that the cause of disease is a mystery or is genetic—beyond our control. Fortunately, this is not so. On the other hand, many, including physicians and informed laymen, are eager for excuses not to face the annoying facts so they can continue to eat in ways that are convenient and agreeable but hazardous to their health.

We Can Stop the Cancer Epidemic Only If We Change Our Diets

If we look at breast cancer as a model to illustrate why cancer incidence has skyrocketed in this century, we can observe that in spite of modern medicine there has been a slow, steady climb in the death rate from breast cancer. Efforts to detect cancer earlier with mammograms and breast exams have not impeded the climb in statistics showing that an increasing number of women are still dying from this cancer. The failure to prevent cancer has exacted an increasing toll: as of 1993 the disease attacks one in eight women in America.

The evidence linking diet to breast cancer has been known for years. As is the case with most other diseases, however, the public is the last to know. In Japan, for example, breast cancer was rare, but Japanese women who migrated to this country soon had the same rate of cancer as American women—at least 400 percent higher than in Japan. We discovered that the decreased rate of cancer was due not to genetics but primarily to the amount of fat in the diet.

In Japan, until about 50 years ago, less than 10 percent of calories came from fat,[25] compared to 40 percent in the American diet, even in the 1940s. Today, however, the Japanese eat more and more meat, fat, and fast foods. Predictably, the rate of breast cancer as well as other cancers in Japan is rapidly increasing.[26] Similar findings have been made within the United States. For instance, studies comparing vegetarian to nonvegetarian groups show much less cancer among vegetarians, especially those avoiding dairy products.[27]

American Children Produce Too Much Estrogen and Androgen

Increased quantities of dietary fat cause an array of negative effects on immune function. The link between higher fat intake and the increasing occurrence of common cancers has been well established for years.[28,29] The link between fat and breast cancer is also explained because it is well known that breast tumors are fueled by estrogens.[30] When women eat a low-fat diet, their estrogen level drops quickly.[31] Fats not only increase the amount of circulating estrogens in the body, but also increase the biologic activity of the estrogen. A heightened estrogen level through life eventually takes its toll—as a cause of menstrual difficulties and increased bleeding, and as an important cause of breast cancer.

This effect of estrogen on the development of breast cancer is also indicated by the fact that women who mature early, as measured by when menstruation begins, face increased risk of developing breast cancer.[32] Sexual maturation is dependent on circulating estrogen levels. Ominously, the onset of menstruation has been occurring at a younger and younger age in western societies during this century.[33] The average age in the United States is now about 12 years. According to the World Health Organization, the average age at which puberty began in 1840 was about 17.[34]

The early development of breast tissue and the early stimulation of this tissue with high levels of estrogen is unprecedented in the history of the human race. This unnatural stimulation of breast tissue occurs before and during the teenage years, setting the groundwork for breast cancer later on. Feeding our children a plant-centered diet predominating in wholesome natural plant foods such as fruits, vegetables, and whole grains is probably the most important thing we can do to prevent them from getting breast cancer as adults. We are finally realizing that the diet we are raised on early in life has profound, far-reaching effects on our later health.

As modern young Japanese have adopted our ways of eating high amounts of fatty foods and more animal products, their age of onset of menses has gradually fallen over the last 50 years from 16 to 12.5 years.[35] The onset of early maturity is an ominous sign both in males and females. As with estrogen in women, heightened levels of androgens in men at a young age set the stage for the development of prostate cancer later on.

Excess Fats Promote Cancer, While Plant Nutrients Protect Us

Comparing various populations around the world, the death rates of most cancers, especially the most common—breast, colon, and prostate—are directly proportional to the dietary fat intake.[36] Dietary fat not only retards the general effectiveness of the immune system, but also encourages the absorption of carcinogens. For example, when the carcinogens in cigarette smoke are absorbed through the lung tissue, the carrier vehicle for their absorption is the fat in the blood. On a low-fat diet the body is less able to absorb and transport carcinogens. Smokers on a high-fat diet have a higher incidence of lung cancer than smokers on a lower fat diet. When we look at the diets of those who contract lung cancer and never smoke, we find a lack of fresh and raw fruits and vegetables.[37]

It is important to note that a diet composed primarily of fresh fruits and fresh vegetables is high in vitamins A, C, and E and high in beta carotene and selenium. These are sometimes referred to as the **antioxidant** nutrients. They are called antioxidants because they have the ability when combined with apoproteins produced by the body to function as scavengers of toxins. They aid in controlling excessive production of free radicals, which are extremely reactive and destructive molecules.

New antioxidant nutrients are discovered every year, but they are not available in food supplements or vitamins. All of these protective nutrients that enable us to remain free of disease are found in the highest quantity in green and yellow plants and fresh fruits. These newly discovered phytochemicals with anticancer activity are being found in increasing numbers in fruits and vegetables. This is one of the hottest areas in nutritional research today.

When we do not eat a diet that obtains most of its calories from fruits and vegetables, we inevitably earn low levels of these antioxidants and protective phytochemicals in our bloodstream. Low blood levels of beta carotene and vitamin C have been linked in multiple studies with increases in cancer mortality, including breast cancer, lung cancer, stomach cancer, and colon cancer.[38] A recent study reported in the medical journal *Nutrition in Cancer* revealed that patients who had a low beta carotene level in their blood in conjunction with a high triglyceride level had a more than tenfold increase in the risk of breast cancer.

High beta carotene and vitamin C levels in the blood are markers for high fruit and vegetable intake, therefore targeting those with a high level of the thousands of other important protective nutrients that travel along with beta carotene. We will never be able to buy them all in a health food store or pharmacy; they can be obtained only by eating large amounts of a variety of fruits and vegetables. Whenever we look at populations who consume high levels of fruits and vegetables, we find reduced levels of cancer and disease in general.[39]

Our present-day diet is responsible for most of the ill health and premature death observed today. In light of the preponderance of scientific evidence available, it would be foolish to consume a diet containing more than 20 percent fat, even though the National Cancer Institute still recommends a diet with no more than 30 percent of calories from fat. Studies indicate that diets drawing 30 percent of calories from fats have negligible effect on cancer incidence.[40] To prevent cancer, fat intake must be reduced to the low levels found in countries with extremely low cancer rates, such as China, where less than 15 percent of calories are derived from fat.

In the massive China Health Study, fat intake in various provinces ranged from 6 to 24 percent of calories. Breast as well as other cancers were proportionally more prevalent as the fat intake increased. Less fat is consumed in the areas of China where cancer incidence is lowest, and this level of fat is much, much lower than what American authorities are recommending. (Our government and our health authorities, like the American Cancer Society and the American Heart Association, recommend a diet proven to cause high levels of cancer and heart disease.)

High-Protein Diets Cause Osteoporosis

The human body is physiologically ill-equipped to handle a diet high in refined foods, animal products, fats, and proteins, without ill effects. Just as heart disease and cancers are strongly related to a high consumption of animal foods, the same can be said of autoimmune illnesses and osteoporosis. Multiple studies have linked osteoporosis not to low calcium intakes, but to diets high in protein, salt, refined sugar, caffeine, and phosphorous contained in soft drinks, all of which cause an excessive loss of calcium in the urine.[41,42,43,44] In fact, populations that consume the highest levels of calcium usually have the highest rates of osteoporosis-related hip fractures.[45] Therefore, osteoporosis should be seen as just another one of the diseases that is linked to our rich, highly refined, high-protein, high-fat, modern diet.

The United States Recommended Dietary Allowance (RDA) for protein is 44 grams for a young woman. This includes a two-fold safety factor, which doubles the minimum requirements as determined by nitrogen balance studies. We do not need to eat any animal foods to meet these protein requirements. Strict vegetarians who eat no animal products get more than enough protein, and they do not need, selectively or scientifically, to mix and match foods to do so.

It is a mistaken notion that we need to eat protein-concentrated foods in order to obtain the eight essential amino acids. A thorough review of the literature on human protein requirements and population studies shows that children and adults grow healthy and strong on vegetable- and complex-carbohydrate-based diets.[46,47] Vegetables that do not contain significant amounts of all eight essential amino acids tend to complement each other even if the amino acids are consumed in separate meals in the same day or as much as 16 hours apart.[48]

The average American woman consumes more than 100 grams of protein per day, which is more than twice the level of our already high RDA. The extra protein that we do not need merely adds stress to the system by increasing the acid tide in our blood-stream after a high-protein meal and forcing the body to deal with excess nitrogenous waste. The stress from excess protein results in premature aging of the kidney and loss of excessive calcium when urinating. This inevitably weakens the bones as we age.

A **negative calcium balance** means more calcium is excreted in the urine than is absorbed via digestion. A positive balance means more calcium is absorbed than is excreted. Studies have shown that when subjects consume more than 75 grams of protein per day, even with a daily calcium intake as high as 1,400 mg, negative calcium balance can result.[49] The continual depletion of our calcium reserves over time from excessive calcium excretion in the urine is the primary cause of osteoporosis. It is the inevitable consequence of consuming the American diet, which is much too high in protein.

Plant foods contain plenty of essential proteins, and you do not have to be a food scientist or dietician to get enough. Any mixture of wholesome plant-based foods consumed in a 24-hour period will supply the body with sufficient amounts. For example, whole wheat bread is 16 percent protein; peanuts, 18 percent; beans, 28 percent; broccoli, 17 percent; and even fresh fruit such as an orange is 5 percent protein. Stop being brainwashed by the false notion that only animal foods contain adequate protein.

Sufficient amounts of protein are obtained when caloric re-quirements are met from wholesome natural vegetable foods. Plant products contain an abundance of protein, without being excessive. How else could the gorilla get to be 800 pounds of muscle, eating solely fruit and leaves? The main point is that we should be concerned about *too much* rather than too little protein. It is ironic that the chief argument used to promote the use of animal products—the idea that they are rich in protein—is a great reason to avoid them.

Increased urinary calcium loss from the conventional high-pro-tein diet also leads to an increased risk of kidney stones and nephrocalcinosis (calcification of kidney tubules). Numerous studies have shown that the formation of kidney stones is directly proportional to the amount of animal protein in the diet.[50] The calcium supplements and increased milk consumption recommended to today's women will further accelerate kidney stone formation and nephrocalcinosis, since more calcium will be filtered through the kidney.

Plant foods are a preferable source of protein also because they do not contain antibiotics, cholesterol, and man-made chemicals that concentrate in animal tissues. Unfortunately, animal foods such as milk, fish, and meat are contaminated with man-made poisons and can contain high levels of pesticides such as PCBs and DDTs. As animals eat the treated feeds and contaminated grains and grasses, they retain the added toxins in their tissues. Animal products contain much higher levels of pesticides than do plant foods.

Animals are fed antibiotics, other drugs, and growth agents. For example, some of the most common drugs used on the farm include **sulfamethazine,** which can cause cancer in laboratory animals and is believed to cause thyroid tumors in humans. As a result of the process of biologic concentration (animals retaining and accumulating poisonous chemicals for a lifetime in their tissues), these chemicals are transmitted to humans when animal products are eaten.

PCBs and DDTs have also been linked to cancer. Women who have breast cancer have a higher concentration of these chemicals in their breast tissues than women who do not have cancer.[51,52] Fish and dairy products are the largest contributors of these toxic products in our diet. Though the highest levels of PCBs are found in fish, they also occur in chicken and red meat. The insecticides DDT and DDE are found mostly in dairy products.

Researchers at the National Cancer Research Center in Tokyo have confirmed other reports that at least ten cancer-causing compounds are known to be released when meat is grilled or fried. Many of the same compounds can be found in cigarette smoke. When these compounds enter breast tissue they can spur cancerous mutations.[53] These compounds, mostly heterocyclic amines, cause cancer by damaging human DNA. The same effect is seen with fish and fowl.

A Natural Plant-Based Diet Is a More Sensible Approach

For ideal nutrition, I recommend a low-fat, lowered-protein, low-sodium diet; one that is high in raw, unrefined carbohydrates. Meals can consist entirely of fruits, vegetables, legumes, whole grains, and raw nuts and seeds used judiciously. This will cut the protein content to less than 75 grams per day. A large salad of green lettuce should be consumed daily.

This ideal diet consists of at least 40 percent of calories from vegetables, including raw vegetables, steamed green vegetables, and cooked starches such as squash and potato. Fruit comprises another 25 percent of the diet, and grains, beans, nuts, and seeds another 25 percent. This diet would derive not more than 15 percent of calories from fat, 10 to 15 percent of calories from protein, and 70 to 75 percent of calories from complex carbohydrate. The fat would come from the natural foods themselves, not from extracted oils.

Refined food products, all sweeteners, added-salt and salted products, as well as soft drinks, coffee, and caffeine drinks would be excluded from an optimal diet. Dairy products would be eliminated or consumed infrequently.

If we look at a sample plant-food menu of approximately 2,000 calories (the caloric intake appropriate for an average adult female), we see that it contains a desirable level of protein, including generous amounts of all the essential amino acids. Even without any nuts or beans, the menu contains much more protein than the RDA.

Breakfast

Oatmeal	(3 cups cooked)
Oranges	(2 medium)
Apple	(1 medium)

Lunch

Vegetable salad, made from lettuce, sprouts, cucumber, carrots, jicama, and lemon	(8 ounces)
Kale	(3 cups, steamed)
Potato	(1 whole, baked)

Snack

Banana	(1 raw)

Dinner

Vegetable salad, made from lettuce, celery, red pepper, carrots, tomato, and lemon	(16 ounces)
Sunflower seeds	(1 ounce)
Broccoli	(16 ounces, steamed)
Brown rice	(2½ cups cooked)

Snack

Grapes	(2 cups)

This sample diet provides 2,095 kilocalories, of which 13 percent come from protein, 74 percent from carbohydrates, and 13 percent from fat. It can be seen from the following analysis that there is plenty of protein in this diet, along with the other essential nutrients. The percent of sodium, rather than being too low, is actually appropriate. The ridiculously high RDA for sodium is reflective of the American norm and is much too high for optimal health.

Nutrient Values and Percent RDA for Selected Nutrients of Preceding Menu

		PERCENT OF RDA
Protein	73.12 grams	149
Tryptophan	851.9 mg	340
Threonine	2,493 mg	554
Isoleucine	3,011 mg	465
Leucine	4,565 mg	480
Lysine	3,185 mg	398
Methionine	1,166 mg	274
Cystine	1,048 mg	246
Phenylalanine	3,124 mg	657
Tyrosine	2,051 mg	437
Valine	3,647 mg	561
Histidine	1,633 mg	296
Calcium	989 mg	123
Magnesium	829.4 mg	296
Phosphorus	1,898 mg	237
Selenium	0.289 mg	525
Vitamin A	8,981 IU	1,122
Thiamine (B_1)	3.429 mg	311
Riboflavin (B_2)	1.960 mg	150
Niacin (B_3)	22.08 mg	147
Pyridoxine (B_6)	4.479 mg	279
Cobalamin (B_{12})	0 μg	0
Folate	844.5 μg	469
Pantothenic acid	8.692 mg	158
Vitamin C	791.2 mg	1,318
Vitamin E	46.28 mg	(No RDA)
A-Tocopherol	66.67 mg	833
Vitamin K	1,376 μg	2,117
Linoleic fat	14.64 grams	299
Iron	25.8 mg	171
Manganese	15.35 mg	438
Potassium	6,728 mg	336
Zinc	12.57 mg	104
Sodium	488 mg	20

On a strict vegetarian diet such as this, the only nutrient that might need to be supplemented is vitamin B_{12}. One B_{12} tablet weekly is sufficient, as the body stores vitamin B_{12} effectively and our needs are very small. Most strict vegetarians do not need to take vitamin B_{12} supplements as their blood level of this nutrient is adequate, probably because of production from bacteria residing within the intestines. I advise people avoiding animal foods to either take a supplement or get a blood test yearly. In a more primitive environment humans on a plant food diet received the small amount of B_{12} needed from bacteria on the foods they ate. Improved hygiene, careful washing, and modern processing destroy this bacteria so, today, it is wise to play it safe by assuring adequate intake.

A compromise diet plan for those desiring to move closer to good nutrition from their present eating habits, but unable to give up animal products, would contain animal foods in very limited quantity. These concentrated foods are such a significant health risk that if they must be consumed, they should be limited to not more than 3.5 to 4 ounces every other day. Even then the animal-based food should be utilized in small quantities, perhaps as a condiment to flavor a vegetable dish or soup. This 3.5 ounces should include all types of animal-based foods.

Another suggestion for those who do not want to restrict themselves to vegetarian foods and who are otherwise in good health would be to eat animal foods such as fish and chicken a few times a month, as in foods for special occasions. Thus one wouldn't have to worry about quantity.

If dramatic improvement in your health is what you have in mind, then dramatic changes must be made in your diet. These changes must be *permanent*. A miraculous recovery from disease, as I see with so many of my patients who adopt these changes, requires dramatic changes in eating habits.

Healthy Diet Food Pyramid
Rational Recommendations for a Healthy Society

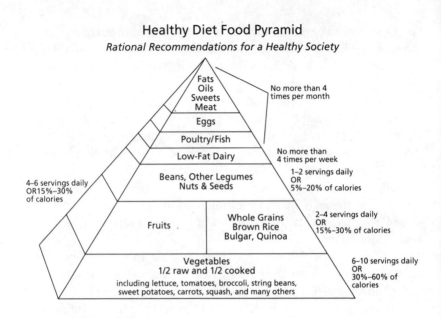

Fats
Oils
Sweets
Meat

No more than 4 times per month

Eggs

Poultry/Fish

Low-Fat Dairy

No more than 4 times per week

Beans, Other Legumes
Nuts & Seeds

1–2 servings daily
OR
5%–20% of calories

4–6 servings daily
OR15%–30%
of calories

Fruits

Whole Grains
Brown Rice
Bulgar, Quinoa

2–4 servings daily
OR
15%–30% of calories

Vegetables
1/2 raw and 1/2 cooked
including lettuce, tomatoes, broccoli, string beans,
sweet potatoes, carrots, squash, and many others

6–10 servings daily
OR
30%–60% of calories

Official Food Guide Pyramid
Issued by the U.S. Department of Agriculture

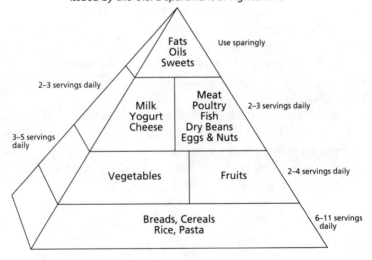

Fats
Oils
Sweets

Use sparingly

2–3 servings daily

Milk
Yogurt
Cheese

Meat
Poultry
Fish
Dry Beans
Eggs & Nuts

2–3 servings daily

3–5 servings
daily

Vegetables

Fruits

2–4 servings daily

Breads, Cereals
Rice, Pasta

6–11 servings
daily

A Healthy Society with Limited Medical Costs Is Possible

Diseases that plague our modern society are reversible if sufficient dietary and environmental stresses are removed from the picture. A good physician can help people recover their health by helping them discover and eradicate all possible impediments to healing.

Reversing disease through nutritional medicine and preventing cancer through diet are the most powerful weapons we have to fight and win the war on cancer and other degenerative illnesses that have taken over our country. Ninety percent of cancers can be stopped before they even start. If just half of the billions of dollars spent on cancer research were spent on educating the public on how to *avoid* disease, we would witness a powerful reduction in the incidence of most chronic diseases. Millions of lives would be saved from cancer.

If we look at heart disease alone, more than $150 billion a year is spent on expensive medical procedures that attempt to remedy the effects of our rich diets. Yet we ignore the reality that heart disease can be totally prevented by a low-fat (less than 15 percent of total calories), plant-based diet. The American Heart Association and the American Cancer Society still recommend a diet with 30 percent of calories from fat.

People are unaware that even 30 percent of calories from fat is an extremely high level when we look at diets consumed throughout human history. Scientific studies show that when this level of fat intake is consumed, there is no improvement in heart disease. On the other hand, it has been shown that at much lower levels of fat intake arterial blockages are easily reversible. When patients who have coronary artery disease are placed on diets containing less than 10 percent of calories from fat, improvement in their condition occurs in a predictable fashion.[54]

The ineffective dietary recommendations from most authorities are comparable to telling a smoker with lung disease that he will be taking care of his disease if he cuts back from three packs a day to merely two. (Unfortunately, these American institutions are misleading the public by recommending diets with a level of fat that has been documented in the scientific literature to actually promote heart disease and cause cancer.)

Instead, our government spends over $20 billion on price supports that benefit the dairy, beef, and veal industry.[55] These dollars are given to farmers to artificially reduce the cost of crops used to feed cows and are also used to advertise and keep the prices down on dairy foods, fowl, and meat. Fruits and vegetables grown primarily for human consumption are specifically excluded from USDA price supports. Out of one pocket we pay billions of our tax dollars to support the production of expensive disease-causing foods. Out of the other pocket we pay medical bills that are too high because our population consumes too much of these rich, disease-causing foods.

Because of animal agriculture's powerful lobbyists, these price supports are not even considered wasteful by our present and past administrations. Worse than wasteful, by keeping fatty foods artifically cheaper, we actually are paying to make our society sicker and keep our health insurance costs high.

Most Americans, though aware of the change in nutritional thinking, have not made substantial changes in their food choices or life-styles. Why? Because most of us are physiologically addicted to food and assume it is difficult to change our diet. We are also confused, uncertain, and have an incomplete picture of how to maintain our health, so we resign ourselves to the way things are. We are unaware of what standards of health are possible for us.

If you have a chronic illness or medical problem, most likely you have been told there are no special diets that will help. This book will put an end to that outmoded, incorrect, and dangerous position, which denies you the chance to regain your health and regain control of your life. Unfortunately, if you try to improve your diet and make changes following the guidelines you have been given from the typical dietician or physician, you will not get better. These recommendations are almost always too liberal to achieve substantial risk reduction or disease reversal. As you will see as we discuss most of the major health problems in detail in later chapters, aggressive nutritional management of specific medical conditions can mean the difference between wellness and a life of chronic illness, multiple medications, and premature aging and death.

Vitamin Pills Will Not Give Us a Healthy Population

It is true that the American public is deficient in certain essential vitamins and minerals, as well as trace elements. Many people are concerned enough about their health to take vitamins, but, unfortunately, this will not have a substantial impact on the wellness of our population. Today almost every medical problem patients are faced with is the result of years of dietary excesses they have consumed, not merely deficiencies.

The message people hear is that it is okay to continue with their present diet, as long as they supplement with vitamin pills or other nutritional supplements. This is a powerful lie, but it is attractive because it is what people in general want to believe. However, you cannot achieve optimal wellness as long as present-day dietary habits continue.

Powerful industrial forces driven by economics, not science, are trying to convince us that it doesn't matter what we eat. Any amount of processed, chemicalized, so-called "food" will allegedly meet our needs as long as we take vitamins, antacids, digestive aids, headache and allergy remedies, and other drugs.

The animal food industry has promoted the use of its products by false nutritional dogma for decades. We have heard this effective misinformation not only from advertisements, but also in the classroom, where it is taught that animal proteins, milk, and dairy foods are essential to good health.

This has occurred as the result of billions of dollars spent by these industries to influence the information we receive. Prevailed upon by powerful lobbyists wielding tremendous economic power, our government has made dietary recommendations that have been at odds with nutritional science for decades. Even with the USDA's latest food pyramid, which de-emphasizes dairy, meat, poultry, and other high-fat foods, the power of the food industry was evident: publication of this pyramid was held up for five years while these food producers negotiated for and won a weaker stance against their products.

These industries financially support and therefore bias the majority of nutritional research carried out by major universities and scientific institutions in this country. For instance, over the last 50 years the largest financial contributors to nutritional research done at Harvard have been the dairy, meat, and sugar industries. Even the American Society for Clinical Nutrition, which pub-

Harvard Department of Nutrition Funding Sources, 1942–1986[56]

American Meat Institute
Armour & Co.
Beatrice Food Co.
Borden Co.
California & Hawaiian Sugar
  Co.
Campbell Soup Co.
Carnation Co.
Coca Cola Co.
Dairy Council of California
Florida Sugar Cane League,
  Inc.
Frito-Lay, Inc.
General Foods
General Mills
Gerber Baby Food Co.
Hartford Foundation (A & P
  Foods)
H. J. Heinz
Hershey Foods
Hunt-Wesson Foods

International Sugar Research
  Foundation
Kellogg Co.
Kraft Corp.
McDonald's Corp.
National Biscuit Co.
National Confectioners
  Association
National Dairy Council
National Dairy Products
National Livestock and Meat
  Board
Oscar Mayer and Co.
Oscar Mayer Foundation
Pet Milk Co.
Pillsbury Co.
Special Dairy Industry Board
Sugar Association, Inc.
Sugar Research Foundation
Swift & Co.
Swift and Co. Foundation
Tuna Research Foundation

lishes the *American Journal of Clinical Nutrition,* discloses on the inside front page of the journal that it is supported by such companies as Coca Cola, Borden, Inc., Nabisco, NutraSweet, and various drug companies.

The result is that establishment nutritional advice does little more than reinforce the dietary errors people prefer to make.

Much of the nutritional information that is given to the public is misleading. Even food labeling is deceptive. Food producers are permitted to use portion size or weight to calculate fat information, which presents a lie to the unsuspecting consumer. For example, is whole milk 4 percent fat? It does contain 4 grams of fat per 100 grams of milk, but since each 100 grams of milk contains 70 calories, and since fat carries 9 calories per gram, whole milk actually gets 50 percent of its calories ($4 \times 9/70$) from fat. Even "low-fat" dairy products still are high-fat foods. The dairy industry always presents nutritional "education" in nutrient/weight terms to hide the fat content of its products.

The meat and fast food industry has even picked up on the dairy industry's mathematical subterfuge. McDonald's "91 percent fat-free hamburger" contains 45 percent of calories from fat.

In spite of the continual onslaught of misinformation, a powerful opposition, and the desire of the majority to want to believe they can consume anything without paying the price, honest nutritional information will eventually reach more and more of the public. This is because we have become such a sickly society that more people are looking for answers.

The facts are that if animal foods are included in the diet in significant quantities, it is impossible to devise a diet consistent with the overwhelming bulk of evidence about food and health in the scientific literature. Society and individuals will pay the price in suffering due to chronic disease and increased rates of premature death.

The diseases most prevalent in our society will never be prevented just by taking vitamin or food supplements. The causes are multifactorial and most significantly the result of eating the wrong type of food. The diseases of affluent societies are virtually unknown in societies of lesser economic strength, which live on natural-food, plant-based diets. When the effects of plant foods are compared to the detrimental effects of animal products, it becomes clear why these "backward" societies have superior health. It is not merely the effects of fiber, vitamins, and minerals in the plant foods that are protective, it is plant foods as a whole.

Preventive Nutrition Is the Same as Nutrition to Reverse Disease

The chicken, fish, and low-fat dairy eating that most people think is healthy for the heart may be a little better than the typical greasy diet, but it is a far cry from a good diet. It will never offer significant protection against or reverse heart disease or cancer. We now have a population of miseducated consumers who think they are on a low-fat diet and wonder why they continue to have high blood pressure and heart disease, not to mention all the other diseases resulting from this outmoded diet. Doctors tell them their illnesses must be genetic or idiopathic (no known cause), which covers up ignorance or inability to improve outcome. The patients are forced to take more medication.

These often ignored points must be emphasized. Even the lower-fat animal products are linked to heart disease, cancer, and auto immune diseases. Also, extracted oils, even the least harmful of them, such as canola or olive oil, still promote obesity and diabetes and even increase the risk of cancer. Keep in mind that when food is not in its natural state (you never saw a jar of oil growing on a tree), it more than likely is a risky food to consume on a regular basis.

If we follow a dietary program that is rich in natural plant foods and eliminates or reduces the intake of refined and overly processed foods and high-protein, high-fat foods, the body remarkably begins to slowly heal itself. The power of your food choices has astonishing effects since food is the most variable and the most substantial external agent that we are in contact with each day.

Fasting, like food selection, is a form of nutritional modification. It has broad biochemical effects on the body. While fasting, the healing process is accelerated. This enables the cells and tissues to clean out the excesses that already exist. Keep in mind, however, that if the message you glean from this book is to fast periodically to give your body a chance to rest and perform internal housecleaning, and yet continue to stress your system between the fasts, you will lose most of the possible benefits.

Rational Recommendations for a Healthy Society

To summarize, general dietary guidelines are suggested here:

1. Eat at least five pieces of fresh fruit a day and a large green salad daily. In addition, a large serving of dark green or yellow vegetable such as broccoli, string beans, or kale (which may be steamed or microwaved if desired) should be eaten daily.
2. Adopt a vegetarian diet, if possible. If you continue to eat animal foods, limit the quantity to less than 3.5 ounces every other day. This includes fish, fowl, meat, and low-fat dairy foods. Unprocessed complex carbohydrates such as baked potatoes, sweet potatoes, rice, and squash should be a daily staple in your diet.
3. Severely limit or eliminate sweets, except for fresh fruit. Fried, salted, pickled, and barbecued foods should also be eliminated from your diet.
4. Drink purified or distilled water, not tap water, which contains chlorine.

If you are seriously interested in your health and longevity, the answers are here for you in this book. But it is pertinent to ask how many people would voluntarily restrict their diet in order to prolong life or lessen the risk of disease? Many believe that people would prefer to satisfy their food desires, rather than live a long life.

When I give presentations on nutrition to hospital staffs or physician groups, a typical statement I receive from someone in the crowd is, "I could never get my patients to do that." This person also is probably thinking, "I don't want to eat like that either."

My response to these doctors is, regardless of the percentage of individuals who would be willing to eat a healthy diet, the least a responsibile physician should do is present the option to those who seek advice and treatment about a significant medical problem. To do less is to sell the patient short. With an accurate presentation, the number of people willing to make significant changes might prove surprising.

In my practice I routinely see patients who are desperately seeking a way to recover their health. It is rare that they aren't willing to make the necessary changes when they are given the opportunity to get well and avoid a lifetime of taking drugs to control symptoms.

3 | Understanding Health and Disease

The ideas presented in this book are centuries old, yet are increasingly supported by new research on human nutrition. It should not be forgotten that today's discoveries and ideas were founded on a long history of scientific effort by physicians who considered nutrition the most critical part of their practice.

As early as 400 B.C. the Greek physician Hippocrates used nutrition as his chief therapy. His favorite healing foods were barley mush, apples, and dates. He paid strict attention to the dietary needs of his patients and stated, "Whoever gives these things [food] no consideration, and is ignorant of them, how can he understand the diseases of man?"

Today the health of our society is poor, specifically because today's physicians know little of human nutrition and the power of optimal nutrition in restoring health. In fact, some of the most respected physicians in history who are remembered because of their success in the treatment of the ill have been all but ignored by the conventional medical community, which bases its practice on giving drugs to the sick.

Isaac Jennings, M.D. (1788–1874),[1] spent 20 years adhering to the regular drugging and bleeding practices of the time, but gradually lost confidence in those procedures and methods. He noticed that he was not helping his patients and found that they did better with fewer drugs. He decided to change his methods. Instead of furnishing his patients with drugs, he gave them placebos, pills and liquids he concocted out of bits of food and water. At the same time, he gave them advice on diet and rest. He often instructed his patients to use the "medicine" for the first week with water and no food. He told them the medicine would not be effective if they did not follow his instructions. He usually continued the plan for a few more days after their next visit. Diseases vanished, and his fame spread. People thought his "medicines" were magical and he became known as the greatest healer of his day.

Early in this century, John Tilden, M.D. (1851–1940), built on the work of other pioneering physicians such as Jennings and devoted his life to teaching the public how to maintain health. He stated,

> Nature returns to normal when enervating habits are given up. There are no "cures" in the sense generally understood. If one has a tobacco heart, what is the remedy? Stop the tobacco of course . . . What will **cure?** Drugs? No! **Removing the cause.** Every so called disease is built within the mind and body by enervating habits. A fast, rest in bed and the giving up of enervating habits, mental and physical, will allow nature to eliminate the accumulated toxin; then, if enervating habits are given up, and rational living habits adopted, health will come back to stay . . . The medical world has been looking for a remedy to cure disease, notwithstanding the obvious fact that nature needs no remedy—she only needs an opportunity to exercise her own prerogative of self-healing.[2]

Herbert Shelton, D.C., N.D. (1895–1985), built on the works of these early medical doctors and wrote prolifically from the 1920s on, in his own self-published magazines and through his publication of 12 books on the subject of health and healing. Dr. Shelton's Health School in San Antonio, Texas, improved and restored the health of more than thirty thousand people through fasting and natural food diets. Both my father, who twice fasted

21 days, and I (who fasted 46 days), were among those thirty thousand patients who fasted at Dr. Shelton's Health School.

To this day, the mainstream of modern medicine and the alternative health-care movement, both fueled by a remedy mentality that dominates our society combined with the financial incentive to make profits selling cures and drugs, has generally ignored this minimalist school of healing. Until recently, little scientific research has been done in this field.

In the last ten years, however, there has been a significant upswing in research on the causes of various diseases. The knowledge gained from these studies, when applied to chronic ailments, will have a major impact on future medical care. It has also lent credence to those "medical heretics" of the past who championed natural food diets and fasting as a means of preventing and treating disease.

The body can heal itself when the proper environment for healing is established and all obstacles to healing, or stressors, are removed. When people live in harmony with their physiological needs, health is the inevitable result. By supplying the organism with its basic requirements—natural unadulterated food, clean water, and appropriate physical, mental, and emotional activities—while simultaneously eliminating all harmful factors and influences, the self-constructing, self-regulating, self-repairing qualities of the body are given full rein. The same innate wisdom that constructed our bodies from two cells at conception is always there to restore the body to health if we let it.

Understanding why we have a health care crisis in this country involves more than looking at political and economic concerns. The primary reason we spend a large proportion of our income on health care is that our population is chronically ill and growing sicker. The "Band-Aid" approach offered by the conventional physician can do little to stop this epidemic of sick people from needing medical care. Unfortunately, legislation will never be able to curtail the runaway medical costs because "disease care," as it should be called, does not lead to a healthier society with fewer medical needs.

Our bodies were designed to function from birth to an un-eventful natural death. But our chance of living in our modern society and then dying from the natural aging process is close to zero. Disease is so much a part of the American way of life that it is considered normal. People do not develop chronic degen-erative illnesses through bad luck. Disease develops through years and years of nutritional and other stresses on the human system. When these causes are sufficiently removed, people can get well, throw away their medications, and avoid unnecessary, expensive, and invasive medical care. It is not aging that makes us sick; it is the stresses we place on ourselves that continue their insidious work over the years and eventually cause damage to the body.

Just because you are ignorant of the harmful stresses that you are placing on your system doesn't make them less injurious. If you drink 6 cups of coffee a day, snort cocaine, and eat fast foods and sweets, it is ludicrous to expect health to evolve from the addition of more drugs in an attempt to lessen the symptoms that arise from the daily abuses that are placed on the body. If the poisoning stops, however, the body has the ability to heal itself and restore normalcy. Clearly, consuming coffee, cocaine, and junk food are examples of practices recognized as obvious stresses to many people, but hundreds of other stressful life-style and dietary practices that are also injurious are generally not recog-nized as so.

Degenerative or chronic disease is earned. Our bodies follow strict biological laws of causation. If we feed ourselves the wrong fuel, or are exposed to toxic substances, if we do not get sufficient rest and sleep, are chronically unhappy or under chronic emo-tional stress, our bodies will inevitably express some malfunction called disease.

These avoidable chronic illnesses encompass almost every con-dition that a doctor sees every day. They include acne and other skin diseases, allergies, asthma, arthritis, diabetes, headaches, heartburn, fatigue, indigestion, psoriasis, high blood pressure, recurrent viral infections, and more. Unfortunately, all patients get when they seek help is more poisons in the form of drugs to consume. These drugs only add to the toxic insults the body must bear, thus further contributing to ill health. Neither the medical community nor the public has understood the simple concept that the body will not function normally if injurious substances are consumed.

It is rare that even years of self-abuse and destruction of the body due to the disease process will cause irreversible damage. When the cause of disease is removed, the rejuvenating effects of the human system are astounding.

Toxicosis Is a Common Cause of Disease

In order to understand the nature of the disease process one must first define **toxicosis**. Toxicosis means nothing more than the retention of elements within our system that are foreign to normal cellular function. It could also refer to the retention of an increased quantity of a substance that would be normal in small amounts but irritating or toxic in higher quantities.

Each cell is like a little factory. It takes in raw materials, processes them into some usable product, and produces waste. This cellular or self-produced waste is called **endogenous** waste. Endogenous wastes are the metabolic wastes produced within our own body, the by-products of cellular metabolism.

Many are familiar with the concept of free radicals, a major endogenous waste whose amount and location in the cell must be tightly controlled to avoid cellular damage. Even the free radical has a positive function within the cell. It is used there as part of the garbage disposal system helping to chew up and destroy other waste products. Only when the amount of free radicals becomes excessive or they escape their normal confines within specific cellular organelles do they become a harmful element.

Exogenous wastes are those toxins taken in from outside the body—usually from our food supply. They include chemicals, pesticides, and other obvious pollutants. These wastes also include excesses of elements that may be nutritive in normal amounts but produce toxic by-products when consumed in larger amounts.

Toxins may also be elaborated from bacteria residing within the digestive tract.

Of course, the body has mechanisms to process and eliminate toxins and protect itself from their damage. This occurs mostly through the breakdown of toxins in the liver and elimination via the kidney. However, the body's ability to process and remove toxic material has many limitations. Given the typical modern diet and environment, our detoxification mechanisms are under stress. They are often chronically unable to keep up with the excessive demand for removal of toxins and other wastes.

Toxins also may be eliminated through the skin and mucous membranes. For example, a skin rash may occur as the body's attempt to rid itself of some offensive substance, or one's nose may produce excessive mucus as the body attempts to channel irritating substances or dead cells through mucosal eliminative channels.

If you were a fireman who entered a burning building and inhaled the acrid smoke, your nose would run, your eyes would tear, and you would begin to cough. Why? Because your body would be making an effort to protect itself from the damage of the toxic smoke.

Your system has means to protect itself from irritants. Is this a sign of illness or of health? Coughing is a sign of health; the body produces a cough as an effort to keep the lungs clear. A healthy body offers a vigorous response when we try to poison it. The body may cough, sneeze, develop a fever or a rash, and even produce mucus or diarrhea in its attempt to rid the system of unwanted retained waste.

It is easy for most people to see how the body can attempt to wash away or push out a toxin such as smoke, but difficult for most to grasp the concept of elimination when there is an invisible irritant coming from within. Waste usually causes no symptoms, just painless cellular damage, unless the body has the means to try to rid itself of the waste. Symptoms occur as the body tries to rid itself of these internalized substances, and excess mucus or inflammatory pain results.

Trying to suppress these symptoms with medication is not a good thing if it enables the body to tolerate more waste products or toxins within it without reacting to them.

In itself, the absence of symptoms is not the same as good health. Like the smoker who continues to inhale noxious smoke on a continuous basis but feels fine, most Americans are poisoning themselves daily in one form or another, yet they feel healthy. Frequently these people feel bad only after they attempt to quit smoking and the body gains the ability to attempt to rid itself of the toxins. Only after quitting smoking does the body begin to repair damage and attempt to remove abnormal cells that have been damaged from years of abuse. So often I hear the complaint, "I felt fine before, but now that I quit smoking, I am coughing and bringing up mucus like I never did before." These symptoms may indicate that the body is moving in the direction of better health.

The absence of symptoms is not indicative of adequate health. Detoxification or rightly directed remedial activities of the body may be uncomfortable or painful, but they always represent a form of withdrawal from an offensive retained element. These same bodily actions may be called into play when the body reacts against an unwanted invader, such as a virus or bacteria and the elaborated toxic products from these microbes.

Occasionally, individuals manifest unusual eliminative pathways that express themselves in troubling symptoms. These may declare themselves in inflammation in almost any body part, but most frequently are observed in the skin and mucous membranes of the nose, throat, sinuses, lungs, vagina, and rectum. For example, vaginitis or prostatitis may be associated with the overgrowth of certain infectious microbes, but in many cases no pathogenic species can be found to account for such symptoms. Physicians are generally not helpful at this point because they have found nothing to treat and kill with drugs so they are unable to offer a solution.

Under these puzzling conditions, it is not unusual for me to see a patient after he or she has visited numerous other physicians to no avail. When the patient undertakes the solutions outlined in this book, and allows the body to finish its rightly directed activity (of detoxification), he or she is soon free from further discomfort. So many symptoms—from unusual skin rashes and joint pains to more infrequent but extremely troublesome proctitis and vulvadynia—are unexplainable by the conventionally trained physician but easily remediable though fasting and natural diet, which allow the body to detoxify.

Exogenous Wastes Typically Come from Food and Drugs

In the first pharmacology lecture that I heard in medical school, the physician impressed on us that all drugs are toxic and we should never forget this. We were taught that medications work because of their pharmacologic properties—properties that enable the substance to interfere with, block, or stimulate an activity of the body. Drugs typically modify the way the body expresses the signs and symptoms of disease, but in chronic disease states, they do not undo the damage or remove the disease.

Of course, medications can be lifesaving in emergencies and in the case of severe infections, such as pneumonia or meningitis. However, the modern drug approaches to chronic degenerative illnesses fail to offer a safe, effective solution for most chronic medical problems.

So medications, alcohol, over-the-counter remedies, and even most herbal remedies (because their primary mode of action is via pharmacologic or toxic effects) can add to the toxic load the body must deal with.

The average person suffers from the effects of toxicosis, or the retention of excessive quantities of waste within the body. This modern type of malnutrition is the result of consuming too much of certain food elements (fat, protein, simple sugars) and too little of others (vitamins, minerals, fiber). When we eat freely of relatively rich foods instead of predominantly natural plant material, we disturb the function of every one of our millions of cells. This results in a buildup of unwanted substances inside and around every cell, contributing to disease.

Improper diet exposes us to many offending substances and is the largest cause of disease. The chief cause of disease in this country is not vitamin or nutrient deficiency. Though specific nutrient deficiencies and imbalances may contribute to the disease process, as does everything from the air we breathe to exposure to chemicals in the home or workplace, their contribution is not so great as the destruction of the body from food-borne toxins and excess nutrients, such as excess fats, proteins, and refined sweeteners.

All Disease Represents an Abnormality in Cellular Function

With the exception of illness caused by direct injury, virulent poisoning, or defects present prior to birth, internal physiology and cellular biochemistry determine an individual's level of health and capabilities. Damage at the cellular level causes groups of cells to function abnormally, eventually leading to chronic disease.

Within the scientific community, the theories of cellular aging, based on advances in cellular biology, explain not only the factors that accelerate the aging of our cells, but also the destructive processes that lead to disease. These mechanisms of cellular damage often express themselves in chronic degenerative illnesses, especially autoimmune diseases, and work to accelerate our death.

In medical research today the **cellular congestion theory** is the leading theory of biologic aging. A few other respectable theories also have advocates in the scientific community. They are presented here because it is likely that no single idea adequately explains all the mechanisms involved in the loss of cellular function that leads to disease or premature aging. When we can comprehend the science supporting many of these most respected theories, we can gain a clearer understanding of cellular function. It then becomes easy to understand how fasting can lead to cellular rejuvenation and why scientific experimentation on animals reveals that fasting prolongs the life span.

The Cellular-Congestion Theory of Aging

Many scientists believe this theory explains why aging occurs. Waste material gathers inside the cell, and eventually accumulates to the point of internal cell damage. The amassing of unwanted and often toxic substances explains the gradual decline in cellular function and therefore body function in general.

The waste products of cellular breakdown and cellular metabolism include excesses and unrestrained free radicals, as well as hundreds of other toxic metabolites. The more stress or the more use demanded from the cell, the more metabolic wastes will be produced.

The Free-Radical Theory of Aging

Free radicals are reactive elements. They contain an unpaired electron, making them chemically reactive. They can break apart other chemical bonds they come in contact with. Free radicals have both negative and positive functions within the cell. Though they are an important toxin, they also function as part of the detoxification machinery of the cell. Cells contain free radicals in order to utilize their reactive and destructive properties to chew up and destroy other wastes. It is only when the production of free radicals becomes excessive and their activity continues outside the confines of the specific areas of the cell that are designed to process waste that free radicals cause cellular damage.

We know now that there are hundreds of other cellular toxins besides free radicals; therefore, it is more precise to include the free-radical theory of aging as part of the cellular-congestion theory.

Since the free-radical theory of aging was proposed in 1956 by Harmon,[3] many attempts have been made to use antioxidants, vitamins, and free-radical-scavenging drugs to see if they extend the life span in lab animals. These interventions have not been effective at extending life spans, though periodic fasting of animals has consistently shown the ability to do so. This failure does not provide strong evidence against the free-radical theory for three reasons: 1) The administered antioxidant may not be distributed to the cellular site of production of the free radical; 2) each antioxidant is specific for a particular free radical species and thus is unlikely to have a global effect; and 3) significant damage to cellular structures, especially the mitochondria, occurs from other nonradical toxins such as malondialdehyde, ceroid, lipofuscin, and other related substances.

On the other hand, fasting (and food restriction in general) has a powerful effect on modulating free-radical production, repairing free-radical damage, and facilitating removal or detoxification of the products of free-radical damage. Fasting aids in the removal of other toxins, and has been shown to maintain the integrity of the cellular structure even at advanced ages.[4] Food restriction also decreases the rate of free-radical generation by reducing the rate of electron transport and oxygen utilization.

The Cross-Linkage Theory of Aging

Tissues in our body, especially collagen, develop cross-links at the cellular level as the tissue ages. These cross-linkages cause tissue to become less elastic and interfere with normal function. Internally produced waste products that are the leading cause of these cross linkages are *intermediate metabolites*. Intermediate metabolites are waste products that increase in quantity as a result of excess nutrient intake, especially excessive protein intake.

When a product the body needs, such as a hormone, is manufactured by the cellular machinery, it is put together by enzymes in numerous steps. The more proteins and other excess raw materials are fed into our system, the more these enzymes will be activated to produce products. Since the body regulates its production of end-products very carefully, it must have a means of controlling this production so that too much product will not be produced. For example, can you imagine if too much insulin was produced?

The body accomplishes this regulation by slowing the activity of the enzymes in the pathway as more fuel (typically protein) is available. As these rate-controlling enzymes slow down, less final product is produced and more partially constructed products, also known as intermediate metabolites, increase in quantity. This explains one clearly defined mechanism via which excess proteins and a few other nutrient precursors are converted into harmful substances within the cells.

Studies have shown that the process of cross-linkage can be retarded in rats by restricting food intake. Overeating and nutrient excesses cause the accumulation of intermediate metabolites, many of which are potent cross-linking agents.[5] When animals are fasted, the aging of collagen is prevented. Fasting inhibits production of cellular intermediates and enables the body either to eliminate such retained wastes or to utilize them as fuel. It was observed that fasting in animals prevented the aging-related stiffening of the blood vessels as well.[6]

This theory of aging is not very different from the cellular-congestion theory. This theory describes further endogenous toxins besides free radicals and shows the powerful effect they can have by cross-linking connective tissue. By combining the above leading theories we can have a more accurate picture of biologic damage on the cellular level.

Genetic-Code-Error Theory of Aging

The genetic code theory is based on the overuse of the cell's genetic machinery, or DNA. The nucleus of the cell contains the architectural blueprint (DNA) for all activity the cell is called on to perform. If the DNA suffers sufficient damage, the cell will not be able to function normally, and could even become cancerous. The more the cell is called on to function, the more the DNA is utilized. Unessential usage of the genetic machinery of the cell encourages more errors to occur in the genetic code and leads to cellular breakdown.

Each cell has a DNA repair team of enzymes that is continually working to repair damage to the cell's vital DNA; however, a cell's ability to repair itself is limited. Free radicals and cellular congestion are known to contribute to DNA damage. This is known as the genetic-code-error theory.

Other theories of aging focus on the function of endocrine glands, growth rate, and rate of immunologic breakdown. Whichever theory we look at can be applied to our model and shows that a nutritionally adequate diet containing no excess nutrients (especially proteins and fats) and no overeating will prolong structure and function at the cellular level.

What these theories all have in common is that we age prematurely when we place our body under stress and drive cellular machinery to overwork in the attempt to process unessential waste. These theories, because they are based on modern scientific knowledge of cells, combined with experimental studies on both animals and humans, indicate that food intake is the most crucial factor that determines aging.

It is remarkable to consider the number of scientific studies illustrating the effect of food restriction on life span. Hundreds of studies have found that in many species dietary restrictions can increase longevity by approxmiately 50 percent. These studies also show that any fat at all on an animal's body has the effect of shortening life span.[7,8,9,10] Fasting animals not only extends their life but also, by blunting most physiologic mechanisms of aging, dismantles immune system imbalances that contribute to disease.

It is also evident that fasting powerfully opposes all the processes that lead to aging at the cellular level. This prolongs life even in healthy individuals. The restorative effects of fasting have been observed in many species of animals (including primates), and have been clinically observed in humans by doctors such as myself who regularly conduct therapeutic fasts.

The Longer the Belt, the Shorter the Life

Many experiments in animals and observational studies in humans show that both severe malnutrition and overnutrition significantly lower resistance to disease. Longevity studies on humans excluding smokers, drinkers, and the chronically ill illustrate that the leanest live the longest.[11] Though thinness is not the only criteria for health, it is undeniable that a person in good health, on a nutritious diet, who is below the average weight has by far the best chance for a long life. The National Institute of Health also reports the same conclusion: when smokers and those with a disease that causes thinness are excluded, the greatest longevity is found in those whose weight is below average.[12]

When the diet is without deficiencies, minimum caloric intake greatly increases resistance to infectious diseases. There are a host of mechanisms that strengthen our immune system and make the "soil" unwelcome for microbes when the body is not overfed. After studying various population groups, including underfed wartime prisoners, researchers have concluded that resistance to disease is highest on what would generally be considered an inadequate diet.[13] It has been noted that when epidemics struck wartime prison camps, the underfed prisoners had a much lower morbidity than their overfed captors.

When we contract a viral infection and lose our appetites, nature is telling us to fast. It is a means the body has of powerfully exciting white blood cell activity and releasing more immune system modulators, such as interferon, thus enabling the body to more quickly and effectively recover.

The best way to guard against nutritional excesses, while still maintaining optimal assimilation of all essential nutrients, is to consume an abundance of natural plant products that are rich in vitamins and minerals. At the same time one must avoid empty-calorie, processed foods, fats, refined carbohydrates, and animal products, which are high in fat and protein and deficient in the nutrients that are most protective to our system.

In the last thousand years, poor societies with constant low caloric intake have had a monotonous, sometimes nutrient-deficient diet, while prosperous, well-nourished societies have blatantly overconsumed calories, fat, and protein. Fortunately, today's modern transportation and refrigeration methods allow us to have an assortment of fresh fruits and vegetables year round, affording us an opportunity to practice a nutrient-rich diet low in fat and empty calories. This has been difficult to achieve in the past. We should take advantage of this opportunity.

Fasting Enhances Immune Responsiveness

Deficiency of nutrients can occur from the consumption of an insufficient diet over a prolonged period of time. Much of our population is indeed deficient in essential plant-derived nutrients because of their overconsumption of fat, protein, and refined carbohydrate. Chronic exposure of experimental animals to diets severely deficient in calories or essential nutrients results in compromised cellular immunity. By contrast, short-term fasting followed by controlled caloric restriction without malnutrition greatly increases longevity and enhances immune responsiveness.

As early as 1911, researchers demonstrated that restricting the diets of animals greatly improved their disease resistance and markedly increased longevity[14,15] as long as the restricted diet was not deficient in vitamins or minerals. Subsequent research has shown that underfeeding reduces the development of both spontaneous and induced tumors in rodents. Specifically, underfeeding enhances cell-mediated immune function and prevents the decrease in immune function associated with aging.

In nonobese humans the immunological response to caloric restriction and weight loss has been studied under conditions of malnutrition, anorexia nervosa, and voluntary fasting. The effect on immune function is marked. Severe chronic malnutrition results in suppression of immune function and increased infections.

Anorexia nervosa patients, if consuming very few calories, develop significant reductions in cellular immunity.[16,17] However, no impairment of immunity is seen until the patients become severely emaciated.[18,19]

In Dr. Anton Keys's classic study of the biology of human starvation, healthy volunteers who fasted repeatedly had a decreased incidence of infection.[20] More recently researchers evaluated the immune competence of patients before and after a 14-day fast and noted enhancement in serum immunoglobulin levels, skin testing response, and the bacteriocidal capacity of monocytes and natural killer T cell activity. These researchers draw a parallel between their findings and the enhanced immune responses seen in experimental animals following fasting.[21]

Fasting is very different from chronic malnutrition. Deficiency disease does not occur as a result of the fast. Rather than suppressing immunity, which is what happens in cases of long-term malnutrition and anorexia, fasting actually does the opposite; it normalizes and enhances immune function.

Our Bodies Follow the Law of Cause and Effect

The body has certain needs. It operates according to strict law and order, not at random. If the laws that govern the body are broken, the body will naturally begin to malfunction and break down. This is really another way of describing what we call disease.

The opposite is health. If you provide the causes of outstanding health, you get outstanding health. If you provide the causes of disease, you get disease. Every level of health, which extends on a spectrum from optimal health and vitality to the disease states of chronic illness, is directly related to and governed by the law of cause and effect.

The general population is bombarded by health information generated by the health profession, drug companies, and food manufacturers, whose intention is to maintain the status quo.

Unfortunately, the average consumer can become more confused than ever. The holistic practitioners, the alternative and complementary physician groups, and the suppliers of vitamins and other natural remedies and treatments add to the giant net of confusion. Everyone claims to have the magic cure. But the sobering facts are undeniable: cure doesn't really exist, so long as the cause is permitted to continue unchecked.

In reality, cure occurs only when the body has rid itself of disease-causing factors and has had a chance to recuperate from their ill effects. What we commonly refer to as being cured is usually the diminishing of symptoms through pharmacology or the removal of diseased tissue through surgery. This is always a short-term solution, does not leave the body in better shape, and sets the body up for a reoccurrence of the same set of symptoms or, in the case of surgery, affliction at a future date elsewhere in the body. The cause, not identified and removed, does not allow the body the chance to heal itself. Healing by means that do not require changing personal habits and taking more responsibility, though always appealing, will commonly fail. Daily I witness the failure of this approach, representative of the failure of modern medicine.

True recovery that does not increase one's later risk of serious illness can result only from positive steps that remove stress from the body. This requires significant personal responsibility and dedication to achieving wellness. Sometimes people really must undertake a fast to recover. Through fasting, individuals are allowed to catch up on elimination of retained waste, thus raising themselves to new levels of superior health. Though most people would rather take pills, potions, and drinks, they often do not make an adequate recovery without the powerful detoxification effect of a total fast.

We all have our inherited weaknesses; genetics always plays a role in the body's form and function. Often this genetic influence determines how disease will express itself as cumulative stresses expose the weakest links in the body's structure. However, these inherited flaws rarely would be given the chance to express themselves if not for disease-causing influences. Improper life-style and primarily improper dietary habits are responsible for the majority of chronic diseases, as well as being the major causes of death in our country. When individuals make aggressive positive changes in their diet, the results can be easily illustrated.

As a physician, it is immensely rewarding to watch people recover from serious disease, as well as routine maladies ranging from obesity to the common cold, through fasting. This is especially true for me since I have witnessed the failure of so many current medical treatments for serious chronic diseases. Medical treatments can be very effective in the short term, but because they do not address the cause of the disease, the person's condition gradually deteriorates.

The laws of nature will never change: it always has been and always will be more effective to remove cause and allow the body's self-reparative powers to have their way than to try to add treatments while cause continues unchecked.

Sleep and Fasting Are the Natural Restorers

Therapeutic fasting can be compared to the recuperative therapy we rely on every night when we sleep in order to charge the body for the next day. Excess stresses, whether from excess consumption of substances or from stressful physical and mental activities, impose negative biological effects on the body. Recuperation through sleep is responsible for rebuilding and preparing the body to handle the increasing demands. Rest and sleep enable the body to recover from the effects of these waking stresses, because the body can concentrate its repair efforts most effectively at this time when fewer demands are placed upon it.

Recuperation takes time, sometimes more time and effort than people recognize. The goal of fasting is to allow time to provide extended physiological rest for the purposes of catching up with recuperative needs generated from the vicious cycle of overactivity, overstimulation, and dietary indiscretions.

If This Diet Is So Healthy, Why Do I Feel So Sick?

If a person truly wants to improve health and rid himself or herself of chronic complaints, it is necessary to recuperate and detoxify. To heal and detoxify, a natural-food, plant-based diet must be followed because natural plant foods not only supply the body with essential nutritive elements needed for optimal function, but also are easy on our organs of digestion and elimination. This diet often does not make a person feel better immediately. Sometimes people initially feel worse when they make positive changes to improve their health.

Before the dietary changes, the digestive tract becomes adjusted to a drier, low-fiber, high-salt diet. After making large changes in one's eating habits, it can take time for the peristaltic waves to adjust themselves to the heavier, higher-fiber, higher-water-content stool, which requires less internal pressure to move along. This may temporarily cause some increased gas and diarrhea, which will improve with time.

Withdrawal symptoms from a prior unhealthy diet are common. Fatigue, headaches, diarrhea, coated tongue, or even a skin rash may occur or intensify at first. These symptoms reflect detoxification and rarely last longer than two weeks.

Occasionally individuals misinterpret detoxification symptoms and think the diet is not working for them, or is lacking in some essential element. Sometimes because they are so misinformed by other physicians, they believe these symptoms to be hypoglycemia or a yeast overgrowth on their tongue. Invariably, though, when they persevere, they soon report that their troubling symptoms have resolved, they feel more energetic, have no more indigestion, and feel and look better than ever before.

We Can Extend Our Productive Lives

People aren't aware that our excessive consumption of dietary fat is a modern phenomenon. Before the Civil War in this country there is hardly any mention of heart attacks in medical books because they were so rare. But now heart attacks are our leading cause of death for both men and women.

Years ago, the rich foods that people consume today were simply unavailable and unaffordable. In the Middle Ages, for example, the kings and queens got fat, and developed gout, diabetes, arthritis, and heart disease, while peasants living in the fields never knew of these afflictions.

The incidence of many chronic diseases and cancers has been increasing steadily in this century. Many years ago a high infant mortality rate, including birth-related deaths, and a higher childhood mortality rate affected statistics concerning life spans. Because infant and early childhood mortality rates were added into the formula, it showed that average Americans lived shorter lives than they do today.

Thanks primarily to better sanitation, modern plumbing with flushing toilets, and refrigeration, life-threatening infectious diseases became less prevalent earlier in this century. This was not due to the advent of antibiotics or vaccinations; this tremendous decline in infections occurred many years before these medicines were introduced.

Many mortality studies have been done on the Seventh-Day Adventists, a conservative Christian group that provides dietary and life style advice to its members. They are prohibited from using tobacco, alcohol, and pork, and are discouraged from consuming meats, fish, eggs, and caffeine-containing beverages. Because the latter items are only discouraged and not prohibited, there is a wide range of consumption of these items. For example, some Adventists never eat meat or eggs, whereas others consume them daily. Furthermore, about one-half join the church as adults and, before converting, these Adventists may have been exposed to a diet high in animal products for most of their lives. If we look at multiple scientific investigations done on this group, we find the following:

1. As a whole, male Adventists live an average of 8.9 years longer than the rest of (nonsmoking) America, and Ad-

ventist women 7.5 years longer (this includes both vegetarian and nonvegetarian Adventists).

Vegetarian Adventists live the longest in proportion to the time they had been on a vegetarian diet.[22] If we extrapolate the results to include those on a vegetarian diet for more than half their lives, more than 13 years are added to the life span, compared to the average nonsmoking American.

2. Egg and meat consumption is strongly associated with all causes of mortality. Dairy product and milk consumption is associated with prostate cancer. The earlier in life that Adventists became vegetarians, the lower their risk of coronary heart disease.[23] These findings are consistent with the findings of numerous epidemiologic investigations, including those done on dairy products and their relation to prostate cancer.[24]

3. All-cause mortality shows a significant negative association with green salad consumption, meaning the more leafy green vegetables consumed in the diet, the longer the life span.[25] This confirms the importance of raw, natural plant foods, the loss of important factors with cooking, and the protective effect of all of the health-giving nutrients they contain.

The conclusion one must make is that animal food consumption is more of a risk factor for an early death than even cigarette smoking. Of course, I am strongly against smoking, but a smoking, lifetime vegetarian probably has a better chance to reach 75 years of age than a nonsmoking, lifetime meat eater.

The opportunity is ours: we cannot rely on modern medicine to give us health and long life. Good health is our own responsibility, and only through accurate information can we protect ourselves and our families.

4 Headaches and Hypoglycemia: Two Misunderstood Conditions

If you regularly suffer from headaches that make you feel as if your head were clamped in a vise, you are not alone. Headaches, including the migraine type, are so widespread that many people consider them a normal occurrence of human existence.

Headaches are our country's number one pain problem and are one of the most common reasons why patients visit physicians. The National Headache Foundation says 45 million Americans suffer from chronic recurring headaches. A recent study has shown that migraine affects 17.6 percent of women and 5.7 percent of men in the United States.[1]

Headaches are a signal that something is wrong. Typically they result from retained toxins in the body. When these metabolic waste products are eliminated, people can regain their long-sought-after freedom from pain.

Most people suffer through their headache attacks using home remedies or over-the-counter medications (on which we spend more than $4 billion each year). When they finally consult a physician, further medication is thrust their way. It is exceedingly rare that the patient will be taught that life-style and diet choices have brought on this problem and that only the removal of these inciting causes can resolve the distress.

Typically, patients are encouraged to become drug dependent, forever popping pills or injecting themselves with drugs in an attempt to control their suffering. This Band-Aid approach will never restore such patients to normalcy. It does not attempt to remove the cause.

Many pain syndromes of undetermined cause have similar biological mechanisms that lead us to feel discomfort. If you are suffering from any type of related pain, by understanding the concepts explained in this chapter you should be able to banish these symptoms from your life forever. The chronic headache patient and the migraine sufferer will be able to throw away their medications and join the ranks of those who rarely—if ever—experience such agony.

Retained Toxins Are the Major Cause of Headaches

The standard theory that tension headaches are caused by widening of the blood vessels and migraines are caused by constriction of the blood vessels has been disproven in recent investigations.[2] The evidence now illustrates the similarities between migraine and other types of headaches rather than the differences. The major cause of both tension headaches and migraines is the retention of toxins or tissue irritants within the central nervous system. These chemical irritants may cause an oversensitivity of nerve tissues to other stimuli.

It has also been shown that tissue waste, such as nitric oxide and other irritating chemicals, can be released from both the nerves and blood vessels in the central nervous system.[3] These recent findings illustrate the biochemical players associated with detoxification in the central nervous system. Withdrawal from toxins either taken orally or self-produced within the body is a form of detoxification. This merely means the body is actively engaged in an effort to lower the levels of waste retained in our cells. Sometimes this release of waste from cells can be painful; nevertheless, it has a positive benefit to the body. Our cells and the tissues they comprise must continually strive to maintain their purity to prevent early cellular degeneration and premature cell death.

One clue to understanding severe headaches is the fact that migraine sufferers are more sensitive to drugs including hallucinogenic agents than people who do not suffer from migraines.[4] This suggests a difference between sufferers and nonsufferers in the blood–brain barrier, or the sensitivity of the brain's surrounding membranes to toxins.

The biochemical mediators causing the pain in so-called tension headache are actually closely related to the causative factors in migraine. Rather than saying that tension headaches and migraines are caused by differing mechanisms, it would be more accurate to see them on a pain and symptom continuum differing only in severity of symptoms and sensitivity of the individual to toxic stimuli and pain-modulation neurotransmitters. The additional symptoms in the migraine such as nausea, visual auras, and dizziness occur simply because the headache is more severe.

For more than 30 years, tension headaches were simplistically believed to be caused by muscle contraction. Now we believe that muscle tension is the response to the pain and not the cause of the headache. Similarly, in migraine, dilation and constriction of the blood vessels follow the onset of pain and do not cause it.

The tension type or muscle-contraction headache is generally less severe than a migraine. It is experienced when the individual is under stress, in contrast to the migraine, which is usually experienced after stressful periods have ended and the body attempts to repair and detoxify. We need not concern ourselves with the minute biochemical differences between migraine-type and so-called tension or muscle-contraction headaches because the biochemical mechanism causing the pain is similar for each, and the treatment described in this chapter is equally effective for both.

The pain of a migraine almost always occurs in the front of the head and is centered on an eye. It is typically accompanied by visual and gastrointestinal disturbances. Essentially, migraines are severe pulsating, or throbbing, headaches, associated with nausea or photophobia.

Many factors may trigger or aggravate an attack of migraine. A common aggravating factor is physical activity. Other common precipitating factors include menstruation, alcohol consumption (especially red wine), too little or too much sleep, a missed meal, or a change in the weather. Certain foods can also trigger migraine in many patients (dietary recommendations will be discussed later).

"Cures" Are Not the Answer

The general medical viewpoint is that migraines cannot be cured, but merely suppressed with drugs. Physicians generally don't hesitate to prescribe medication for a person to take for the rest of his or her life. The common medical practice of giving drugs (which are all toxic) to treat the ill effects of retained toxins, without attempting to determine and remove causative factors, is a misguided approach illustrative of the overall inadequacy of today's health care system. Fortunately, I can take my patients off these drugs when they learn how to adopt healthful diets and life-style practices that are much more effective at preventing such attacks.

During the first pharmacology lecture I attended in medical school, the instructor admonished us never to forget that all drugs are toxic. Indeed, many of their effects on the body are obtained because these substances are toxins that interfere with or poison the body's natural activity. Besides contributing to the body's toxic overload and leading to overall deterioration in health, it is well recognized that the medications used to treat migraines are a crucially important factor in perpetuating future attacks. Drugs that are used for headaches—such as acetaminophen (Tylenol), barbiturates, codeine, and ergotamine—all cause headaches to recur on a rebound basis as these toxins begin to wash out of the nervous system. Then, in order to temporarily lessen the pain, headache sufferers take more of these tissue poisons, only to excite another attack in the near future, thus maintaining the patient on a drugging merry-go-round.

The use of medication, even in quantities as low as ten aspirin tablets per week, can be the cause of a chronic daily headache

79

syndrome.[5] The best thing a physician caring for headache patients can do is withdraw their medication. One medical study found that stopping all treatments and pain medication actually *decreased* headache frequency and intensity in the subjects by more than 50 percent.[6]

Besides the typical toxic drugs that physicians routinely prescribe, toxins such as alcohol, lead, arsenic, morphine, carbon monoxide, pesticides, and noxious fumes can cause severe headaches.

Likewise, other unhealthy practices—drinking coffee and soft drinks, eating sweets and other nutritionless foods—contribute to the problem. Even drinking milk can add to our discomfort, as it frequently contains multiple antibiotics given to the cow.

Most individuals in our modern society are dealing with the ingestion of drugs and other chemical toxins almost daily and are continually, and sometimes painfully, attempting to detoxify. Taking further poisons into the system to prevent the painful elimination of wastes merely perpetuates the problem and allows headaches to recur more frequently.

Just as we can "cure" the coffee drinker's headache by giving him or her more coffee to stop the withdrawal or elimination of the retained toxins associated with caffeine consumption, so, too, can we "cure" the heroin addict's withdrawal symptoms by giving him or her more heroin or by substituting methadone. We can "cure" the headache or migraine sufferer's problems by giving him narcotics, or by prescribing Esgic, Ergostat, Bellergal, Cafergot, Excedrin, Fiorinal, Vanquish, or Wigaine, which contain either caffeine, ergotamine, or barbiturates.

These approaches, although widely employed and accepted, do not remove the cause and, in fact, perpetuate the problem they attempt to solve. Prescribing such medications merely temporarily curtails symptoms of withdrawal, not much different from the pusher on the street corner, selling his wares to the addicts who must suffer pain should they not continue to take their narcotics. Headache patients should never be given opiates, barbiturates, or caffeine (which are found in many headache remedies) as these substances will always make the problem worse in the long run.

Many other medications also cause headaches, both the garden variety tension headache as well as migraines. These drugs include those used for angina and high blood pressure, as well as estrogen-containing birth control pills and estrogen hormone replacement therapy, often prescribed after menopause.

When migraine and tension headache patients are placed on low-protein, natural plant-based diets, with no refined sweets of any type, they almost all recover within a month, never needing medication or further treatments to control their condition.

What to Do and What Not to Do If You Are a Headache Sufferer

Most people mistake feeling good for health. But anything that quickly makes you feel good is likely to be harmful to your health. Often, in order to recover your health you may have to temporarily feel bad so your body can cleanse itself of an offensive substance. Cocaine may make a person temporarily feel better, but you would not argue that cocaine use is a healthful practice. Anything that rapidly takes away symptoms of ill health or makes you feel stimulated is likely to be a health risk. *Superior health must be earned through healthful living.* The road to optimal health through removal of cause may take a little longer, but the result you earn will be everlasting.

Drugs to relieve pain are rarely necessary if headache sufferers are allowed to fast and detoxify at the first sign of headache symptoms. Patients trying to detoxify and eliminate dependency on medication often find it useful to retire to a dark room and use ice compresses or a tight ice wrap around the head to reduce pain. An alternative can be to stand in a hot shower with hot water beating on the painful area. In addition, biofeedback techniques such as progressive relaxation and self-hypnosis can often be helpful to these patients.

Commonly, though, such techniques are not needed because the headache sufferers have quickly eliminated their headaches through the nutritional approach described here. By the time biofeedback methods are learned, they are no longer necessary. If the person still suffers from headaches during the first week after the diet is changed, I find cold and pressure to be most effective and practical.

Many individuals with migraine can obtain effective relief by simply applying an elastic band around the head, securing it with Velcro, and inserting rubber discs for added local pressure over the areas of maximum pain. An investigational study utilizing a 2-inch elastic band approximately 25 inches long with Velcro at each end illustrated impressive results with this non-drug approach for relief. Firm rubber discs the thickness of a finger and a little over an inch in diameter were employed. Patients were instructed to place these discs under the elastic headband over the area of maximum pain. Almost every patient in the study reported benefit. Twenty-three patients used the band for a total of 69 headaches. Forty of the headaches were relieved by more than 80 percent and 15 headaches improved by more then 50 percent.[7]

One should be warned that when one is not continuing to ingest harmful food substances, the body will often use this opportunity to detoxify, and that may initiate another headache. This is the time when the patient must try to use physical modalities—such as cold compresses, seeking rest in a dark room, banding with Velcro, and biofeedback—and at all costs avoid the use of further medication. Employing such mechanical approaches and avoiding medication will enable the headache sufferer to avoid taking toxic drugs, which will interfere with the body's ability to manifest a complete recovery through nutritional intervention.

Headache can be exacerbated by not eating. The reason is that not eating triggers withdrawal symptoms as the body begins to detoxify and get rid of retained toxins. Remember: For a short time you must feel bad so that for a long time you can feel good.

Obviously, some headaches may result from brain tumors, meningitis, tuberculosis, hypertension, head injuries, and diseases of the eyes, nose, throat, teeth, and ears. Such conditions are rare, however. Allergic conditions and chronic sinusitis are also uncommon causes of headache. Persistent severe headaches that do not respond within a few days of fasting should always be further evaluated by a physician. The onset of a severe headache like one never experienced before, especially in an older person, should also be properly evaluated by a physician.

Eating Right Can Eliminate Migraines

Headaches can worsen around menses, and have a tendency to run in families. Sometimes headaches are caused by food allergies, and anyone with severe migraines should avoid foods that have been noted to trigger headaches. Salted foods are frequently noted as a trigger, as are chocolate, cheese, ice cream, nuts, eggs, banana, herring, fatty foods, citrus fruits, NutraSweet (aspartame), MSG (monosodium glutamate), nitrates (often present in processed meats), and concentrated sweets. MSG and aspartame have similar chemical structures, and frequently those who react to one also react to the other. Alcohol is a frequent offender, not only because it can act directly to trigger headaches but also because it contains chemical amines added as flavorings that are potent migraine producers.

Since MSG can cause severe headaches and migraines,[8,9] as well as other symptoms, foods containing this ingredient should be totally avoided by headache sufferers and possibly challenged (reintroduced as a test) at a later date when the person is doing well and is headache-free. Delayed symptoms may occur even 72 hours after MSG is ingested, so it is sometimes difficult to trace the symptoms back to the offending substance. Some researchers estimate that only 1 to 2 percent of the population is sensitive to MSG, while others believe the figure is closer to 25 percent.[10, 11]

Unfortunately, if you are trying to rely on food labels to disclose the presence of a substance that you wish to avoid, you will frequently be deceived. Since MSG and other food additives can sneak into so many processed and packaged foods, it is best to avoid all such food items completely if you are a chronic headache sufferer. Since such avoidance is extremely difficult for most people, the table below may be helpful for those sensitive to MSG.

Food Additives That Always Contain MSG[12]

Monosodium glutamate	Yeast nutrient
Hydrolyzed protein	Autolyzed yeast
Hydrolyzed vegetable protein	Textured vegetable protein
Sodium caseinate	Calcium caseinate
Yeast extract	Yeast food
Hydrolyzed oat flour	

Food Additives That Often Contain MSG

Malt extract	Malt flavoring
Bouillon	Natural flavoring
Barley malt	Natural beef flavoring
Broth	Natural chicken flavoring
Stock	Natural pork flavoring
Flavoring	Seasonings

A high-protein diet is one of the most common reasons people suffer from chronic migraines. Protein breakdown and digestion causes the production of multiple toxins, especially nitrogenous wastes, many of which easily cross the blood–brain barrier. Humans are designed by nature to consume a low-protein diet; they lack the equipment of a large liver to detoxify uric acid and other proteinaceous wastes. We frequently suffer unknowingly from our modern dietary practices because our bodies are not adapted to handle the foods we eat.

A basic plan to rid one's life of headaches is to start a low-protein, plant-based diet specifically designed to avoid the foods listed below, as well as all caffeine-containing products. The severe migraine sufferer should strictly adhere to the food plan described here until a definite recovery is achieved. Later, when the individual has fully recovered, the diet can be expanded to include some of the prohibited fruits and vegetables to see whether or not they cause a problem.

To start, headache sufferers should withhold all medication, including oral contraceptive pills (utilizing another method to prevent pregnancy). They must stop consuming all herbal preparations, food supplements, tea, soft drinks, coffee, and all caffeinated beverages. Once these steps have been accomplished, it is time to follow the rest of the program:

1. Avoid all salt and MSG, including soy sauce, oriental foods, canned soups, sauerkraut, pickles, and sauces or processed foods that may contain salt or other preservatives and artificial flavorings.
2. Avoid all sweets, including honey, maple syrup, dried fruit, or sweet fruit juice.
3. Eat no animal foods, including beef, pork, fish, poultry, eggs, and dairy food. If you add a small amount of animal food on occasion after a recovery has been achieved, keep the portion size down to less than 4 ounces (the size of a deck of cards) and stick to chicken, turkey, or beef, avoiding fish, ham, and all canned, cured, or processed meats, or meat prepared with tenderizer.
4. At the beginning, avoid most fruits and all fruit juices. Bananas, citrus fruit, pineapple, apples, applesauce, pears, apricots, avocados, cherries, figs, fruit cocktails, papaya, passion fruit, peaches, plums, and raisins should all be avoided. Melon and grapes are the only fruits allowed. These may be eaten in a small amount before breakfast or as a snack. Once a recovery is achieved, more fruits may gradually be included in the diet. Bananas and citrus fruits should be saved for last.
5. Avoid nuts, seeds, and all legumes, including pole or broad beans, lima or fave beans, lentils, snow peas, navy beans, pea pods, garbanzo beans, onions, or olives. Once

a recovery has been achieved, a small amount of beans—
less than 4 ounces daily—can usually be tolerated.
6. Avoid all dairy products, especially cheese sauce and salad
   dressings containing milk derivatives such as whey.
7. Avoid all yeast-containing products, including brewer's
   yeast.

Here is a sample diet for migraine patients in the first phase
(Phase I) of their recovery.

Breakfast
Small piece of melon
Oatmeal or other whole grain hot cereal or yeast-free
   whole grain bread

Lunch
Large green salad (no dressing except 1 teaspoon olive oil
   permitted)
Corn, sweet potato, white potato, brown rice, steamed
   carrots
Bunch of grapes

Dinner
Small salad
Steamed green vegetable such as broccoli, artichoke, kale,
   cabbage, or asparagus
Starchy vegetable or grain such as butternut or acorn
   squash, potato, corn, millet, quinoa, rice, or pasta. To-
   mato sauce made without salt is OK

As stated earlier, sometimes headaches continue for a few days
while the body is still eliminating retained wastes, but usually this
diet results in the quick elimination of the patient's problems.
   Once a definite recovery has been achieved and the patient is
free of headaches for one month, some of the prohibited foods
may be added back to the diet. Add one food every few days,

particularly avoiding any food that clearly precipitates an attack.

Start with fresh fruits, reintroducing them into the diet a little at a time. Then begin to include legumes, and then a small amount of nuts or seeds. If the person swings back to his or her former eating habits and begins consuming a significant quantity of animal-based, high-protein foods or highly salted processed foods, the headaches invariably return.

Headache Sufferers Easily Recover

Taking care of patients with recurrent headaches or migraines is probably the most rewarding patient interaction I experience on close to a daily basis because these patients typically recover very quickly. A couple of examples will suffice, as there is not much to say about headache case histories, except that if the patients do what I tell them to do, their headaches quickly disappear. So often, before the patients have been referred to me, they have seen a neurologist or other physician, who besides treating them with the typical drugs has ordered or recommended an MRI scan of the brain. I typically tell patients to hold off on these expensive tests for a few days while they follow my program and, invariably, they feel well in a short period of time.

Kate was a 42-year-old woman with a 20-year history of severe and frequent migraine headaches. When she first came to see me she was taking Fiorinal and Repan on a regular basis as prescribed for her condition. She was also taking Deconsal for sinusitis and allergic rhinitis.

Kate started the migraine-reversal diet, and at the next visit three weeks later reported that her headaches as well as her chronic sinus condition had completely cleared. She no longer needed medications. She experienced only one further episode, the day after the first visit, and has had no further symptoms.

Kate later told me that for the first time in her life she was able to fast during Yom Kippur (the Jewish holiday of atonement). Prior to this year she experienced an excruciating headache and other hypoglycemic symptoms whenever she attempted to fast.

Nancy, a 34-year-old woman, also had recurrent migraine headaches. They were especially troublesome and severe around her menstrual periods. Her headaches were accompanied by nausea and a desire to vomit. She was using Xanax, and Repan as prescribed by her former physician. Nancy started a Phase I diet and was tapered off the medications. Her headaches quickly disappeared, and she has not had another problem with headaches since instigating this program. An added benefit was that her periods were no longer painful.

These patients did not need to stay on the Phase I diet for long. Other foods were quickly introduced, and they remained symptom-free.

Occasionally when people's symptoms are very severe and they wish to accelerate their recovery, they can begin with a two- to three-day fast, followed by the recommended diet. If the headaches do not resolve completely from their lives after following the plan described here, a longer, medically supervised fast for a more adequate detoxification must be considered.

Occasionally a patient with a severe condition may require a more prolonged fast to clear out the retained wastes that are causing the problem. For example, when Gordon came to see me he had already consulted with dozens of renowned physicians for his severe headaches and facial pain. He was taking 16 Percocet tablets (a powerful narcotic) and 2 Klonopin tablets (a tranquilizer) daily. His headache, accompanied by piercing pain, never left him for a minute. If he did not take high doses of narcotics, the pain was unbearable and he had no normal existence. Because of his severe problem, he was forced to leave his job. He and his family were in financial distress. Besides unsuccessfully trying every headache medication in the book, he had undergone facial and sinus surgery, temporal artery bypass, and injections with nerve-blocking medications, all without improvement to his excruciating condition.

After starting a simple plant-based diet, I slowly weaned Gordon off his medications over a month-long period. His facial pain was very severe without the narcotics and I placed him on a fast as soon as possible. Within a few days of fasting all his pain resolved. So that he could more completely detoxify, I extended his fast for an additional two weeks. He is now back working and for the first time in 20 years is pain-free.

Our bodies try hard to keep us healthy. When disease-causing stresses are removed, the natural healing and self-repairing powers of the body begin to work unhindered. This self-repair and self-cleansing occurs most efficiently in sleep and when the body is no longer working hard or digesting food. During these times the system can more effectively devote its efforts to housecleaning and the elimination of retained wastes.

Conventional Thinking Often Results in an Oversimplified Diagnosis of Hypoglycemia

Hypoglycemia means low blood sugar (the terms "blood glucose" and "blood sugar" are equivalent). Frequently I encounter patients who are convinced, based either on their own interpretation of their symptoms or on the diagnosis of a physician, that they have a disorder caused by swings in blood sugar levels.

Their complaints usually include one or more of the following: weakness, fatigue, headaches, abdominal pain, mental confusion, clouded vision, rapid heart beat, anxiety, sweating, shaking, and incoordination. These symptoms typically appear three to four hours after eating, especially when eating has been delayed or a meal has been skipped. Since these symptoms occur at the time when one's glucose level is at its lowest, the patient or physician attributes the problem to low blood sugar—thus the diagnosis of hypoglycemia.

There are two basic types of hypoclycemia: **fasting hypoglycemia** and **reactive** or **functional hypoglycemia**.

Fasting hypoglycemia is generally due to serious and potentially life-threatening disorders such as insulin-secreting tumors or advanced liver dysfunction. Other causes of fasting hypoglycemia include drugs used for diabetes, alcohol, advanced renal failure, and hormonal deficits. All these conditions are relatively rare. In them, blood sugar levels can plummet dangerously, resulting in profound weakness and even coma and death. Obviously, individuals with this condition require urgent medical care.

Reactive or **functional hypoglycemia** is the second type of hypoglycemia and the common type that is the focus of this chapter. This type of hypoglycemia results in problematic symptoms, though the blood sugar levels do *not* drop to dangerously low levels. The prevalence of this condition is unknown, largely because there is no widely accepted criteria for its diagnosis.

Some physicians have taken the position that reactive hypoglycemia is very common and is the cause of innumerable ills. When encountering patients with symptoms suggestive of reactive hypoglycemia, many of these physicians advise them to eat frequent meals of high-protein foods. This is usually effective at reducing or controlling the symptoms.

Are these common symptoms, experienced by many, caused by low blood sugar? Is a high-protein diet the best way to control this troublesome condition? My answer to both these questions is an emphatic **no.**

There is much misinformation that surrounds the issue of hypoglycemia. As with many other health ailments, health professionals tend to lump patients with many different medical problems they can't solve into a convenient diagnosis. I will attempt to help clarify this confusing issue.

Glucose Metabolism—A Finely Tuned Balancing Act

Our brain and body tissues require glucose for survival. Without adequate glucose circulating throughout our bloodstream and other tissues we would die. Thus the prevention of hypoglycemia is critical to our survival.

The two major hormones that control our circulating glucose level are **glucagon** and **insulin.** Basically, insulin drives the blood sugar down and glucagon raises it. Insulin drives the glucose out of the bloodstream and into the cells. Other hormones secreted to maintain our blood glucose level when we are not eating include **epinephrine, cortisol,** and **growth hormone.** The prevention of hypoglycemia between meals requires an intact liver and the appropriate regulatory hormones to control it.

The Glucose Tolerance Test

Reactive hypoglycemia cannot be accurately diagnosed merely by a glucose tolerance test. First, understand what occurs during a glucose tolerance test: Before any readings take place, patients must fast for 12 hours. They then ingest 100 grams of sugar. Every hour afterwards, for five hours, blood is drawn and the glucose level is monitored.

In the first hour after glucose ingestion, the patient's glucose level is high. The body takes a bit of time to react to the very large quantity of glucose it has ingested, but is then stimulated to secrete an unnaturally large amount of insulin to rapidly lower the exceedingly high level of glucose that has entered the bloodstream. As insulin is secreted, the glucose level drops. Plasma glucose concentrations often reach nadirs of less than 50 mg (and sometimes less than 40) in normal people who experience no symptoms. However, when a person's glucose level drops to 60 mg or less (the lower range of normal) and they start to experience symptoms, a doctor labels that person **hypoglycemic.** This is overly simplistic.

The glucose tolerance test is notoriously unreliable. It is an artificial and stressful stimulation and it can be expected that many normal people will get sick from this experience. When a large dose of concentrated sugar (glucose) is consumed after an overnight fast, we can expect it to produce a sudden surge in insulin secretion in response to the unnatural stress on the pancreas. This situation (consuming a large amount of refined sugar) might make many of us feel ill, but this is not indicative of disease. Consuming such a quantity of refined carbohydrate is always stressful to our system and should definitely be avoided.

Other reactions and the release of additional counter-regulatory hormones also occur to compensate for the insulin surge. Therefore, it is not only the lowered blood sugar that makes a person feel ill. Besides that, the majority of patients diagnosed by physicians as having hypoglycemia never had blood glucose levels below 60 mg on their glucose tolerance tests when they experienced symptoms.

In general, consuming concentrated sugars is stressful to the system. Besides generating wide swings in blood sugar, the consumption of sweets can deplete the body of nutritional reserves needed for optimal immune and endocrine function. Refined sugar products and other concentrated sweets can cause excessive fluctuations of insulin and other hormones that can cause symptoms in healthy people. This does not mean they have hypoglycemia.

A more reliable way for individuals to discern if their symptoms correspond with low levels of glucose in their blood is to go to the doctor's office or laboratory at the exact moment when they begin experiencing their symptoms, and get their blood tested. People usually find that their blood sugar levels are not unusually low at the time. In fact, it is very rare for them to find that their blood sugar is low when they are symptomatic.

But what about individuals who feel terribly ill at the same time their blood sugar is low? Does this mean that their symptoms are caused by low blood sugar? Not necessarily. They may be caused by other biological processes that cause discomfort and occur in the system at the same time the blood sugar drops. **Gluconeogenesis** is the process by which we maintain our glucose levels between meals by breaking down stored reserves of noncarbohydrate tissues (primarily protein). During gluconeogenesis (which occurs when blood glucose levels are low), urea and other nitrogenous wastes are dumped into the bloodstream as the body's tissues are broken down. These products can make a person feel ill. Therefore, it is not merely low glucose levels that can cause the ill feeling; there are a number of other factors involved.

Most of the symptoms individuals complain of when they think they have hypoglycemia would not occur if low blood sugar alone was responsible. Though weakness, hunger, and sweating are typical symptoms of low blood sugar, visual disturbance, mental confusion, headaches, and anxiety are not. These latter symptoms result from decreased activity of the central nervous system and do not occur simply because of low blood sugar. Headaches and anxiety, for example, do not occur in "fasting hypoglycemia," such as when a diabetic is overmedicated by mistake, unless the person also has an autonomic neuropathy (nerve damage) that blunts the release of epinephrine.

Usually individuals who manifest these complaints when their blood sugar is low are not accurately described or diagnosed as hypoglycemic, and the standard treatment that follows is not satisfactory. We must first comprehend the true nature of these symptoms before we can understand the most effective way to help the individual who suffers with this problem.

Recurrent Headaches—A Close Relative of Hypoglycemia

Troubling symptoms such as headaches, mental confusion, and anxiety that accompany a low blood sugar reading have biochemical similarities with the more common tension or migraine headaches. It is incorrect to believe that low glucose is the cause, though it may seem that way. Certainly it is easy to see why people think this, because the headache occurs at the time when the glucose dips when eating is delayed or a meal is skipped.

Assume you were drinking 12 cups of coffee every day. How would you feel if you suddenly stopped drinking it? Terrible, right? You would have severe headaches because when the caffeine is withdrawn the body attempts to detoxify or remove the buildup of this noxious substance. This is called withdrawal, or detoxification. Suppose you were addicted to high doses of heroin. Would you feel better if you tried to quit? Of course not. You would experience weakness, trembling, abdominal pain, and severe headaches. Detoxification from most noxious substances results in symptoms much like those noted by individuals who claim they have hypoglycemia.

If a heavy coffee drinker skips a meal, a severe headache will probably occur. Heavy coffee drinkers who delay breakfast for a few hours will also experience mental fatigue, headaches, and confusion. Those who are not addicted to coffee will generally not suffer when breakfast is delayed. Are the headaches experienced by caffeine addicts caused by low blood sugar? They occurred only when the blood sugar was at its lowest point, but clearly these are manifestations of withdrawal or detoxification that occur because we skip or delay eating and the body eliminates retained noxious material most effectively at this time. The body takes the opportunity to accomplish self-cleaning, or detoxification, when it is not busy digesting and assimilating food and nutrients.

Likewise, the symptoms of so-called hypoglycemia are most often related to withdrawal or detoxification. Resolution of this condition is best accomplished by methods that allow the body to lower its toxic load. To call these symptoms hypoglycemia shows a gross oversimplification of what is occurring and illustrates an insufficient understanding of body chemistry.

There are hundreds of other toxins our body may be exposed to on a daily basis. When we skip a meal, delay eating, or fast, the body almost immediately begins to detoxify and clean itself of waste. Withdrawal from any one or many of these non-nutritive substances retained in our tissues can generate a sickly feeling of weakness, confusion, or headaches.

When patients undergo therapeutic fasts, blood sugar levels below 50 mg per deciliter are not uncommon. As the fasters' blood sugars dip to low levels, they may experience weakness and lethargy. Though these patients occasionally experience headaches, the headaches always resolve with continuation of the fast. This is the body's way of telling us the elimination of the toxins causing the symptoms has been completed. Even if the blood sugar levels continue to fall, the headaches do not recur. This illustrates that these symptoms were not the result of low blood sugar, but were caused by other processes that were occurring simultaneously with the lowering of blood glucose.

Those who fast after following low-protein, plant-based diets have less discomfort and are less likely to have a headache during the early stages of a fast. This is because withdrawal from proteinaceous or nitrogenous wastes is the chief culprit that precipitates headaches and sickly feelings.

High-protein diets and medications can control symptoms of so-called hypoglycemia in the same way continued coffee drinking controls symptoms of caffeine withdrawal. Individuals with these conditions can completely recover without resorting to dangerous high-protein diets or medication to control symptoms. Treatments and high-protein diets give only temporary relief as they do not address the cause.

Problems with Protein

In the United States and many other industrialized countries, a diet high in protein is thought to be health promoting. Unfortunately, most people indoctrinated with this notion in their youth still cling to this outdated and potentially dangerous misconception. In reality, high-protein diets are linked with the development of serious diseases including cancer, heart disease, osteoporosis, rheumatoid arthritis, lupus, renal insufficiency, and kidney stones.

As human animals we are not biologically adapted to a high-protein diet. Metabolically there is little difference between humans and the great apes, who are predominantly vegetarians. Like the ape, we are not adapted to function optimally on diets that are high in protein and fat. Therefore, we suffer the consequences of heart attacks, cancer, autoimmune illness, and so on when we consume a diet ill-adapted to our basic constitution.

The misunderstanding of human protein requirements began 70 years ago when two scientists published the results of a study that showed that rats fed vegetable protein grew more slowly than rats fed animal protein. Today, we have to interpret this information much differently. First of all, we now know that humans and rats have different protein requirements and that people can get all the protein they need from plant sources. More important, we now have found that rats that grow and mature the quickest *die earliest*. Not only is rapid growth a poor indicator of the value of a food, but foods that promote rapid growth in animals and humans are the precise foods that promote premature aging of our body and even cancer.

With all species the longer an animal takes to reach maturity, the longer it lives. We know, for example, that women who mature earlier as measured by their age of puberty have the highest risk of breast cancer. So another reason to avoid high-protein foods is that they promote premature growth and maturity.

The average American consumes about 150 grams of protein a day—about five times the amount actually needed. This excess protein, not to mention the fat that accompanies it, is extremely damaging. So what does this have to do with headaches and hypoglycemia? Plenty. Consuming excess protein produces certain toxins, by-products of animal food digestion, which enter our bloodstream. These toxins have the ability to cause central nervous system symptoms, such as mental confusion and headaches. The effects of these toxins become most noticeable when the digestive tract is not busy digesting and glucose levels are low. It is under these conditions that nitrogenous wastes are effectively mobilized.

Since the American diet contains more protein than we need, the liver attempts to break down the excess and excrete it in the form of urea via the kidneys. The level of urea is measurable in the blood with a blood test called **BUN,** or blood urea nitrogen. Urea is one irritating substance that results from consuming excess protein. However, there are many other toxic by-products of protein metabolism besides urea that are not so easily measurable in the bloodstream. Researchers are finding that many of these other by-products of protein digestion have a powerful toxic effect on the brain, and can cause mental fatigue and confusion as their levels rise in the body.

The liver is the major organ of detoxification and it is especially when the detoxification pathways in the liver are compromised that we see an increased likelihood that individuals will suffer from the toxic effects of their high-protein diets. A good way to illustrate the effect excess protein has on cerebral (brain) function is to look at patients with diseased livers. Patients with advanced stages of liver failure who cannot adequately metabolize excess dietary proteins develop a change in mental function, drowsiness, confusion, and disorientation. They may eventually become markedly confused before lapsing into a coma. Dietary proteins, especially the ones containing sulfated amino acids and aromatic amino acids—from the proteins contained in animal products—must be significantly curtailed in patients with liver disease. This is the established treatment for this condition. Without restricting animal proteins, their disease and mental condition will significantly worsen.

A crucial point to keep in mind here is that there are about 14 other toxins besides urea that are breakdown products of protein metabolism. Even though urea is the only one we can inexpensively measure in the bloodstream at this time, the other protein-related toxins are more responsible than urea for the mentally confused state we see in cirrhotic individuals.

Uric acid and other potentially harmful nitrogenous wastes such as ammonia increase in our body when we consume excessive protein. Vegetable proteins generate less ammonia and other harmful wastes and are less acid-forming as well.

The typical American diet, which is high in protein, especially animal proteins, results in a high level of retained nitrogenous wastes and metabolic toxins that have to be either eliminated or stored for future removal. When we give the body the opportunity, it will attempt to eliminate such toxins. Sometimes corresponding painful symptoms of mental fatigue, jitters, and headaches will occur during this detoxification period.

Hypoglycemic persons can recover and no longer need to be addicted to high-protein diets to control their symptoms. Individuals with a lower level of retained wastes (especially proteinaceous wastes) in their systems will not suffer from the symptoms generally regarded as hypoglycemic when their blood sugar dips. They will recover because their bodies no longer need to discharge nitrogenous wastes and other retained toxins in between meals.

A Different (and Natural) Solution for Hypoglycemia

So what should you do if you believe you have hypoglycemia?

1. Stop consuming foods that contain refined carbohydrates and simple sugars. These foods will be absorbed into the body rapidly and force an excessive insulin response. On the other hand, high-fiber foods slow the absorption of nutrients and glucose and therefore do not cause an excessive insulin response.

   Especially avoid sweets other than fresh fruit. Fruit not only contains trace elements needed for the adequate metabolism of its contents, but also has its sugars bound in fiber, which causes the sugars to be absorbed into the bloodstream more slowly.

2. Stop consuming high-protein animal foods. Instead, replace them with vegetables, fresh fruits, legumes, and unrefined grain products.

3. Avoid all soft drinks, coffee, tea, artificially flavored or colored foods, and food additives. Avoid alcohol and caffeinated beverages as they exaggerate hypoglycemia and result in withdrawal symptoms exacerbated during the low blood sugar nadir.

4. Consume some food every two or three hours during the first few weeks to minimize symptoms while your body is suffering from "withdrawal" from your previously rich diet.

5. If necessary, eat a small amount of high-protein plant foods such as beans or nuts and seeds with each meal for the first month or so when you eliminate animal proteins

from your diet to minimize the initial withdrawal symptoms from an animal-protein-based diet.

After conforming to the above guidelines, people find they can return to a wholesome plant-based diet with no further symptoms of so-called hypoglycemia. With time, more than 95 percent of patients with these complaints never have another symptom. If, after a reasonable amount of time, one still gets uncomfortable symptoms before the next meal, he or she should consider a fast to permanently resolve the condition. Fasting quickly and predictably resolves symptoms of hypoglycemia because it so effectively allows the body to lower the level of retained toxins, which can cause tissue irritation.

Occasionally individuals will have unusually severe symptoms of hypoglycemia. Sometimes they will feel so bad that they are unable to function or live a normal life. The approach described here has enabled my patients to recover when all other methods had failed them.

Samantha, a woman in her early thirties, had such severe hypoglycemic symptoms that she was forced to quit her job. She had seen multiple physicians and had undergone numerous tests. Her fasting glucose level ranged from the forties to 70. She eventually became so weak that she was admitted to the hospital for further evaluation. During her hospitalization, her doctors could find nothing seriously wrong with her except for unexplained hypoglycemic symtoms. Though still so weak she could barely walk, Samantha was discharged from the hospital with instructions to remain on a high-protein diet.

When Samantha first came to see me she was eating eggs, beef, turkey, ham, and cheese every two hours all day and most of the night. She accompanied each meal with a glass of milk. She could not walk for even two blocks. She was physically disabled, forced to quit her nursing job, and too debilitated to seek any other line of work.

At the start, I maintained Samantha's eating schedule of every two hours but substituted plant protein for animal protein. Gradually, over the next eight weeks, we eliminated all animal protein. Instead, Samantha ate tofu, beans, lentils, chick peas, lima beans, and pumpkin and sunflower seeds, and increased her intake of green vegetables. Over the next few months we made gradual dietary adjustments so that her symptoms would not worsen. Her illness was so severe that I thought she would need to undergo a prolonged fast to completely recover. I was wrong. She made steady progress. The severe incapacitating symptoms slowly resolved, and she soon reported that she had a good energy level. She was able to walk 30 blocks without a problem and has had no further symptoms. She is now back to work, living a normal life.

You, too, can forever rid yourself from troublesome symptoms, merely by adopting the best nutritional program, one that is more appropriately designed for your natural genetic tendencies: a plant-centered, natural-food diet.

5 The Road Back to a Healthy Heart—the Natural Way

Cardiovascular Disease and High Blood Pressure Can Be Safely Reversed Without Medications, Angioplasty, or Bypass Surgery

Cardiovascular disease is our nation's number one killer! The gradual clogging, hardening, and damage done to the interior walls of our blood vessels are the primary cause of heart attacks and strokes. This process of atherosclerosis, or hardening of the arteries, also results in poor circulation to the extremities, the brain, and other organs. Ailments such as senile dementia, leg pain (intermittent claudication), and even erectile impotence have their origin in atherosclerosis.

Yet, by means of appropriate dietary approaches, heart disease, blood vessel blockages, and high blood pressure can all be prevented and *reversed* after they occur. As with other debilitating problems, these diseases are commonly the result of a high-fat, high-protein, highly refined diet that is ill-adapted to the needs of our species. The accumulation of fatty plaque on the inner walls of our blood vessels begins early in childhood and progresses gradually through life due to modern-day dietary practices.

High blood pressure is the result of blood vessels that are relatively inelastic due to deposits of plaque. Fatty plaque causes blood vessels to become stiff and weak. Such stiffened vessels lose their elasticity and are more likely to tear or rupture from high blood pressure, thereby causing a stroke or heart attack. Taking medication to lower blood pressure does nothing to reverse or remove the atherosclerotic blood vessel disease.

Half of the population over 65 years of age has high blood pressure. It is the leading reason for prescription medication in the country today.[1] In numerous countries, however, where the diet is not rich in fats and protein, and is high in fiber and fresh produce, high blood pressure is virtually nonexistent.[2,3] Atherosclerotic disease of the blood vessels and heart occurs only in parts of the world where high-fat and high-protein diets are consumed, but heart attacks are virtually unknown in societies that follow natural plant-based diets.[4,5]

As this chapter will show, fasting, followed by an appropriate diet, gives people a choice that can enable them to discard their hypertension medication and live in good health.

Current Treatments for Cardiovascular Disease Are Ineffective and Dangerous

Current treatments for clogged arteries include medication to lower blood pressure and cholesterol levels, bypass surgery, balloon angioplasty, and arthrectomy. Although surgical procedures can relieve the symptoms of chest pain (angina), they result in little or no improvement in how long a patient survives. In addition, these treatments are dangerous. Some patients die during surgery or soon afterwards.

In numerous cases, various drugs are prescribed to lower cholesterol levels and relieve chest pain. These drugs come with their own inherent dangers. Cholesterol-lowering drugs may slightly reduce the risk of future cardiac events, but, because of other undesirable metabolic effects, they increase the cause of death from other causes. Side effects and costs are considerable as well.

Cholesterol-lowering drugs are well known for their liver toxicity and can also cause life-threatening reactions such as muscle breakdown and acute renal failure.[6]

Drugs for angina relieve the pain, but they do not reduce the chance of a heart attack or sudden death. All together, medications are minimally effective or ineffective in prolonging life because they do not halt the underlying disease process (atherosclerosis). Furthermore, as the patients are left with the false impression they are now OK, their disease-causing life-style is indirectly encouraged, since they rely on medication for symptomatic relief or lowering of blood pressure. This lessens the essential importance of meaningful dietary change. It is interesting to note that the well-known Helsinki heart trial showed no significant difference in the total death rate between the group treated with a cholesterol-lowering drug and the group given a placebo.[7]

Today, the use of cardiac diagnostic and treatment procedures is growing at an alarming rate. More than 300,000 bypass surgeries costing more than $40,000 each are performed each year. Huge profits are involved, but bypass surgery rarely prolongs life. If the patient manages to get through surgery and its aftermath in the hospital, alive and without complications, the subsequent death rate is about 2 to 4 percent per year thereafter. Of patients who have comparable levels of heart disease, 2 to 4 percent die each year without surgery. The general death rate is the same in both instances, with or without surgical intervention.[8]

While high-tech methods aim to reduce symptoms, they do not address the underlying *cause* of the disease. People inevitably get sicker and die unnecessary cardiovascular deaths.

Compare this to therapeutic fasting and natural diet, which not only quickly relieve symptoms, but also strip the body of its cardiovascular risks. This natural approach results in the prolongation of life and the avoidance of cardiac death.

If every patient with cardiovascular disease were placed on a fast, followed by a truly low-fat (less than 10 percent of calories consumed), natural plant-based diet, millions of lives could be saved. Added benefits would include the savings of billions of dollars in practically worthless medications, unnecessary testing, invasive procedures, and surgeries.

Bypass surgery is under increasing criticism by the medical community, and most doctors are aware that bypass surgery fails to save lives. Bypass is not only unproven but also has been *disproven*. Even the *Journal of the American Medical Association* reported that more than 125,000 of these procedures are done for inappropriate reasons each year.[9] The Office of Technology Assessment of the U.S. Congress has also criticized the unproven character of bypass surgery.[10]

Women are more at risk from these procedures than men. It is not generally known that the in-hospital death rate for bypass surgery is 4.45 percent for women and 3.33 percent for men.[11] Bypass surgery is also associated with a 13 percent rate of post-operative complications, including heart attacks, strokes, bleeding, kidney failure, and infections.

In almost every heart bypass patient, some brain injury occurs from the time spent on the heart-lung machine.[12] It is believed that 15 to 44 percent of those who survive such surgery suffer permanent brain damage, detectable as minor degrees of intellectual impairment, memory loss, sleep disturbance, and personality change.[13,14,15]

There are some critics who say that bypass surgery has been shown to have a slight survival advantage over medical treatment for those patients with a severe blockage of their left main coronary artery or severe triple vessel disease. Not denying this, we must consider that this situation affects only a small percentage of patients undergoing bypass. More important, this slight survival advantage is observed only if we compare such treated patients to other patients on medication who live on the disease-accelerating American diet. I believe the combination of fasting and a natural, zero-cholesterol diet would offer even patients with advanced cardiac disease a significant survival benefit.

Surgery should and can be avoided. Even if there is some short-term reduction in symptoms, atherosclerosis then accelerates in arteries after they have been subjected to bypass or angioplasty: the plaques grow faster after surgery.[16] The arteries treated by both angioplasty, arthrectomy, and bypass often reclog within a short period of time. Approximately one third of arteries dilated by angioplasty clog up again within four to six months.[17]

Angioplasty has never been tested in a prospective trial against medications only, so doctors are in disagreement about its value despite its widespread use. Since the native blood vessel has now been interfered with, the new blockage that so often soon reappears is now more difficult to treat with nutritional methods. This restenosis (return of the treated blockage) is not the same as the original atherosclerosis. Restenosis is a new disease created by doctors (called iatrogenic disease), and it is not controlled by the same processes that control the disease process in untampered-with coronary arteries. Lipid-lowering measures, smoking cessation, dietary change, weight loss, and decreasing blood pressure do not prevent restenosis or have a significant effect on its reversal.

Balloon dilatation is a risky crap shoot, 30–40 percent of patients will need to go back again for more invasive interventions. Another problem is that balloon angioplasty is a self-referred procedure in general and incredibly compelling to perform from the cardiologist's perspective. We need to keep in mind that angioplasty has some significant adverse outcomes, including myocardial infarction (heart attack), cerebrovascular accident (stroke), and death.

Doctors should really think twice about doing interventions that could potentially kill the patient or lead to significant disability. When we compare the potential benefits and risks of these traditional though invasive procedures to the nutrition interventions described in this book, these procedures look foolish. This situation is especially tragic because aggressive nutritional approaches are typically not even discussed with patients.

Though high-tech methods, new drugs, and advances in surgical techniques aim to reduce symptoms, the underlying cause of disease—a disease-causing diet—goes completely ignored or is addressed with inadequate and improper advice. The patients inevitably get sicker and sicker.

Natural Methods Are Both Safer and More Effective

The encouraging news is that we now know heart disease is both preventable and reversible. Every cardiac patient should be made aware of this. Unfortunately, the general public, as well as many physicians, is not aware of the fact that coronary blockages, high blood pressure, and angina can be reversed without drugs or surgery.

For years, there has been a small number of avant-garde physicians who have been using very low fat diets to reverse cardiovascular disease. These nutritional approaches are much safer than conventional treatments; they are more effective, and, most important, they prolong life. Now, when a healthy diet is combined with controlled therapeutic fasting, we can offer even cardiac patients with advanced disease a noninvasive, safe, effective approach that can literally rejuvenate their entire cardiovascular system in a short period of time.

Before I explain this approach, let's look at some of the recent studies of diet and cardiovascular health. Both interventional studies and large epidemiologic (population-based) studies conclusively document that certain diets promote cardiovascular disease, and that other diet-styles can both prevent and reverse it.

The Lifestyle Heart Trial

One of the most important recent studies on the effect of diet on heart disease is the Lifestyle Heart Trial, conceived by Dr. Dean Ornish.[18] It demonstrated that blockages in blood vessels were effectively reversed when patients combined a plant-based zero-cholesterol diet with exercise and stress management, and that the most severely blocked arteries showed the most improvement.

This interventional study, conducted on patients with documented coronary artery disease, split patients into two separate groups, the **control** group and the **intervention** group.

The control group was placed on the American Heart Association's (step 2) recommended diet, similar to the diet recommended by the American Diabetic Association for diabetics. This diet suggests cutting out butter and choosing chicken or fish instead of red meat, although a limited amount of red meat is still allowed. This change of eating habits reduces fat intake from the American norm of 40 percent of calories from fat to 30 percent. It keeps cholesterol intake to less than 200 mg daily. This control group was also advised to exercise and stop smoking. All patients had cardiac catheterization before beginning the study, and one year later the cardiac catheterizations were repeated to document the effect of the intervention.

Many were surprised to find that the majority of subjects in this control group did not improve. They carefully followed standard medical advice (Step 2: American Heart Association Diet) to stop smoking, to exercise, and to cut down on fat by eating chicken (without the skin) and fish. Yet the followup cardiac catheterizations on this group showed that a majority had a *worsened* cardiac status after one year.

This result is not surprising since we know from numerous other medical studies that the usual advice (recommendations of the American Heart Association and most physicians) does not halt the progression of heart disease; it merely slows down the rate at which a patient's condition will worsen.

Imagine if you came to me with a breathing problem stemming from a three-pack-a-day smoking habit. If I said to you, "Don't worry, I can help you—just cut back from smoking three packs to two, and you will get better," would you expect good results? Studies have now conclusively documented that the typical dietary advice doesn't work: the level of fat and cholesterol permitted is still much too high to allow improvement. People only *think* they are on low-fat diets.

In comparison, the intervention group in the Lifestyle Heart Trial was placed on a truly low fat diet, with less than 10 percent of calories derived from fat. To achieve this ratio, they ate without restriction in quantity from plant foods such as fresh fruits, vegetables, legumes, and grains. A limited amount of egg whites and nonfat milk or yogurt was allowed. Dr. Ornish found reversal in atherosclerotic plaque in 82 percent of coronary heart disease patients from this intervention group after one year on the vegetarian diet, combined with light exercise and stress management.

The important findings emerging from this study have served to change conventional thinking about reversing heart disease. The findings include:

1. Age has nothing to do with atherosclerotic plaque reversal; even elderly persons show impressive improvements.
2. Individuals do not have to lower their cholesterol levels to below 150 to get reversal. Compliance with the program was what was related to the reversal, not the degree or number to which the cholesterol level dropped.
3. Even arteries that have been totally blocked for years open up.

Dr. Ornish has astutely noted in a January 1994 interview in *Visions Magazine*:

Conventional wisdom is that small, gradual changes are easy and big, rapid changes are hard. If anything, we have found that the reverse may be true. When you make small, gradual changes, you get the worst of both worlds. You get a sense of deprivation, because you're not getting to eat or to do everything that you enjoy, but you're not making changes big enough to be of much benefit. Your cholesterol, your blood pressure or your weight don't come down enough. Your chest pain doesn't get better. Worst of all, if you have heart disease, according to not only our study, but those conducted by the American Heart Association and National Cholesterol Education Program, in every one of those studies where people made moderate changes, the majority of those patients get worse.

As Dr. Ornish states, his study is only one of several that document that the standard recommendations (following a diet in which 30 percent of calories come from fat) still allows the progression of heart disease.[19] Yet research studies, such as the Lifestyle Heart Trial and others, document that heart disease is reversible with vegetarian diets.[20,21,22] These studies were designed after it was noted in numerous population-based studies that cardiovascular deaths were virtually nonexistent in rural populations consuming vegetarian diets. Additionally, it is noted by researchers that deaths from heart disease increase gradually as populations gradually increase their consumption of animal-based foods.[23]

The China-Oxford-Cornell Project

The most famous of the epidemiologic studies on diet and health is the China-Oxford-Cornell Project (called the Grand Prix of epidemiology[24]). This study clearly documented that the diseases that affect and kill most Americans are unusual in rural China. Dr. T. Colin Campbell, the leader of the China Project, stated:

> The average protein intake from animal sources in the United States is 70 percent. In China, only 7 percent comes from animal sources, so there is a tremendous difference between the two countries. But in spite of the low levels of protein intake from animal sources in China, if they add just a little bit (animal protein) to the diet, the cholesterol levels start going up, heart disease starts going up, and cancer increases. This tends to suggest that it doesn't take much animal protein to start changing cholesterol levels and consequently have the risk of heart disease and cancer.[25]

The more animal protein consumed, the higher the cardiovascular risk. In fact, those Chinese who ate the most protein (even fish) had the highest rate of heart disease, cancer, and diabetes.

The Dangerous Recommendations of the American Heart Association

All animal foods are rich in fat and protein and deficient in fiber and antioxidant nutrients that protect against heart disease and cancer. Many studies looking at populations consuming 30 percent of calories from fat illustrate a substantial amount of cardiovascular deaths, and all studies done on populations that consume under 15 percent of calories from fat show that heart disease and diabetes are virtually nonexistent.[26,27,28]

Standard medical advice for controlling heart disease and lowering cholesterol levels is usually to switch from beef and pork to chicken, fish, and skimmed-milk dairy products. Unfortunately, this advice does not work. Cardiac disease invariably worsens.

A recent investigation analyzed the data from 16 different trials evaluating the possible benefit of the American Heart Association Step 1 diet. It concluded that this advice is essentially worthless, and that the "Step 1 diet produced no significant gains in cholesterol reduction at any of several time points."[29]

Once again it is important to note that a diet in which fat calories are lowered to 30 percent is still too heavy in animal-based foods, which cause heart disease. A diet that includes salad oils, chicken, fish, and dairy foods is a high-fat diet for our species. Though the average American consumes even more fat (40 percent of calories) than the American Heart Association guidelines, dropping the fat ratio to 30 percent is simply not enough.

These standard recommendations still allow the progression of atherosclerosis because the diet is still too high in cholesterol, too deficient in antioxidants and fiber, and too abundant in animal-based protein. Since the cholesterol levels in chicken and fish are equivalent to those in beef and port, dieters' cholesterol levels do not show a meaningful change. Studies in which chicken or fish was substituted for beef in human subjects have shown no significant difference in blood cholesterol level regardless of the choice of animal flesh.[30,31]

Dr. John McDougall, the author of *The McDougall Plan* and

other books, has pointed out on numerous occasions that the cholesterol and fat content of the American diet is so far in excess of the amount necessary to cause heart disease that relatively small increases or reductions are unimportant. Once one has exceeded the amount of dietary cholesterol needed to cause illness (as little as 100 mg cholesterol per day), any more makes little appreciable difference.[32] For example, the egg industry can publish studies that show that the addition of an egg to an otherwise high-cholesterol diet has little impact on raising cholesterol levels further. However, when people on a no-cholesterol diet are fed even one egg a day, their cholesterol level rises considerably.[33]

My intention here is to explain why the conventional recommendations and treatments fail at truly removing the risk of cardiovascular disease, as a preliminary to presenting an approach that is predictably effective even in the most advanced cases.

Fasting: A Powerful Means to Reverse Cardiovascular Disease

In addition to aggressive dietary changes as described above, a physician-supervised therapeutic fast can be utilized to bring a patient to a new level of cardiac safety. Fasting, in conjunction with optimal nutrition before and after the fast, offers the ability to undo the damage done to the body by the rich diets of modern societies. Through therapeutic fasting a patient is able to reverse a cardiac condition quickly, without the need for invasive medical procedures. The results I have seen in patients using this approach have been spectacular.

There are some cardiac conditions in which patients are at such risk that it is imperative the blockages in the arteries be quickly diminished. People who have been told they need bypass surgery or angioplasty, as well as those with angina at low workloads, are prime candidates for therapeutic fasting. Fasting allows the body actually to remove the plaque from within the blood vessels and to heal itself in the shortest amount of time.

There is always a choice. One can be put to sleep in the

operating room, have one's sternum split and chest pried and stretched open, have a heart-lung machine pump blood while the heart's action is stopped, and risk death or a decline in mental ability—all this for results that will not significantly increase the life span. Or one can combine a fast with a healthy plant-based diet that can facilitate a recovery and a new lease on life.

I find most patients who choose to get well via aggressive nutritional approaches are angry that their other physicians did not give them this option before they were told they must have bypass or angioplasty. Patients must be given this choice of a very low-fat vegetarian diet and fasting because it is safer, cheaper, less invasive, and more effective at extending the patient's life. Anything less is selling the patient short.

The deplorable state of cardiovascular health we have in our nation and the current ineffective methods for treating heart disease should not continue. The general public must learn how to challenge heart disease as the nation's number one killer. Those suffering from the ravages of heart disease must be told that there is a safe, less invasive way to get relief and prolong their lives. A plant-based diet in conjunction with a properly conducted fast most often leads to a total recovery or a vast improvement in hypertension and angina.

This method of treating cardiac patients is not new. Studies in the medical literature on fasting as a treatment for heart disease began in the 1960s. Over the years, reports of improvements in cardiac status from fasting documented consistent benefits ranging from reducing blood pressure to alleviating angina and congestive heart failure.[34,35,36]

Dietary restriction has for a long time been considered an effective approach to many chronic diseases. After World War II studies of populations that underwent semi-starvaton during wartime rekindled physician interest.

It is interesting to note the diseases that were reported to be quite rare during the period of semistarvation. Among these were coronary artery disease, hypertension, congestive heart failure, gastric and duodenal ulcers, appendicitis, nephritis, cholecystitis, hepatitis, diabetes, hyperthyroidism, allergic states, upper respiratory infections, and rheumatic fever. Only with improvement of the nutritional state did some of these return to their former prominence as causes for hospitalization.[37] Autopsy studies during the years following World War II showed that clinical atherosclerotic disease became extremely rare as well. This demonstrates the cleansing of the lipid component in plaques. The reabsorption of atheromas has also been well studied and documented with wasting diseases such as cancer,[38,39] and also with dietary restrictions and fasting in nonhuman primates.[40]

It is such a simple concept, yet so far away from the consciousness of today's modern physician, to simply allow the body to reabsorb the blood vessel blockages with an aggressive nutritional approach. When we utilize this knowledge and combine an extremely low fat diet with fasting, the potential to clear the blockages within the blood vessels is maximized. Patients can expect better results than when following the strict diet alone.

Chelation Therapy Compared

Chelation involves the intravenous infusion of EDTA (ethylenediaminetetraaceticacid) and is promoted as a nonsurgical alternative to angioplasty or bypass. Its value and positive effects are controversial. EDTA is a powerful drug that is used to treat mineral poisoning because it pulls minerals such as calcium and lead out of the body.

Chelation therapy for atherosclerotic disease is similar to other temporizing measures. It might relieve pain and improve circulation temporarily through vasodilation, but there is no solid evidence that it can remove the atheromas or plaque lining the vessel walls; nor does it decrease one's risk of sudden death. I have seen many patients who have received hundreds of chelation treatments without improvement and then watched their chest pain quickly resolve with one fast.

A perfect example is George, a 69-year-old man with a history of diabetes, hypertension, high cholesterol, and angina. He had already experienced one heart attack. When I saw him for the first time he was using four different medications: Tenormin, Lopid, Orinase, and a nitroglycerin patch. After 175 chelation treatments, and while following what he thought was a very low fat diet suggested to him by his prior physicians, he continued to suffer chest pain and chest pressure. These symptoms were felt even while he was resting.

I explained in detail my treatment plan and I immediately stopped the medication he was taking to lower his blood sugar level. Following my advice, he took care to adhere to a "less-than-10-percent-of-calories-from-fat, zero-cholesterol" diet. He returned to my office two weeks later.

At this time his blood sugar level was better controlled than it had been at his first visit, when he was still on medication. My next step was to taper the other medications, leaving only the nitroglycerin patch two weeks prior to the start of his fast.

When he arrived for his fast, his weight was down to 175 pounds from 182 pounds. Because he was still experiencing chest pressure without the nitroglycerin patch during the early part of the fast, I maintained the patch for the first week of fasting. By week 2, he was experiencing no further angina and I was able to discontinue the nitroglycerin patch without further problems.

George fasted a total of 19 days. For 4 additional days I gradually introduced a diet of fresh fruit and vegetables before sending him home. His weight was 151 pounds.

A month later he called me excitedly while vacationing in Florida. He was now walking more than two miles a day, off all medication, and angina-free. He was no longer diabetic, either; his blood sugar levels were well within the normal range.

I have now seen enough patients who have undergone chelation with no benefit to conclude that this therapy is just like other drug treatments, only minimally helpful, if at all, and more expensive. These same patients, when introduced to aggressive dietary changes, had dramatic positive responses. The fact that a cardiac patient must continue the chelation treatments indefinitely and receive hundreds of treatments to maintain its supposed effect also indicates it is not removing the disease.

The few well-designed double-blinded studies that have addressed the efficacy of chelation for atherosclerotic disease have not found evidence that chelation offers benefit over dietary intervention.[41,42] Since both the EDTA-treated and the placebo-treated groups fared the same, the authors concluded that the beneficial effects were closely correlated with motivational encouragement from the physicians, improved diet, and more exercise, rather than from the therapy itself. Other carefully done, randomized, double-blind trials also concluded that no therapeutic effect of chelation could be demonstrated.[43,44]

Certainly, further studies will be done to evaluate chelation. Attractive as it may be for those people looking for an effortless cure, chelation still does not remove the cause of disease—high saturated fat and cholesterol-containing foods. The primary treatment must be dietary, with a zero-cholesterol diet. Then, as an adjunctive measure, fasting is the quickest and most effective complement to diet to accelerate recovery.

Fasting Quickly Lowers Blood Pressure As It Extends Life

For a person with advanced cardiovascular disease, fasting can not only begin to reverse the damage caused by years of improper eating, but also rapidly decrease the risk of sudden death from a heart attack or stroke.

First of all, fasting rapidly and effectively lowers blood pressure without medication. In most cases this effect is permanent if the person maintains the correct eating pattern after the fast. A period of therapeutic fasting will lower blood pressure even in severe hypertension. Many of my patients who have had difficulty controlling hypertension utilizing combinations of three or four different drugs have had their blood pressure decrease into the normal range through fasting. Moreover, blood pressure generally remains low upon the reintroduction of food if they continue to follow the recommended diet.

Greg came to me after suffering from repeated transient ischemic attacks. These "mini-strokes" can be a warning sign that a serious and life-threatening stroke is likely to occur. His blood pressure was difficult to control with diet alone, so the dose of his blood pressure medication was increased and another medication was added. Though taking the highest suggested dose of two blood-pressure-lowering agents, he continued to have elevated blood pressure and still suffered from headaches and visual disturbances. Fearful he would experience a stroke, I advised him to undergo a fast as soon as possible. At the start of his fast and while medicated, his blood pressure was 150/90, and he weighed in at 236 pounds.

Greg fasted for 12 days. I tapered his medication until he was receiving no medications by day 4. At that time his blood pressure dropped to 132/90. At the end of the fast his blood pressure was 110/78 and his weight had dropped to 216 pounds.

At the time of his follow-up visit to my office a few weeks later, his pressure was 108/76. It has continued to remain in the low, normal range with no medication, as he continues to adhere to a proper diet.

The medical literature confirms these findings. In a study of 683 obese patients of whom 48 percent had high blood pressure, it was noted that rarely did these patients continue to have high blood pressure after two to four days of fasting.[45] This phenomenon has been consistently noted with both obese and nonobese patients.[46,47]

In Dr. Alan Goldhamer's ongoing study of fasting and hypertension, so far 51 people with high blood pressure have been fasted an average of 11.2 days. The average blood pressure when these individuals began fasting was 151.8/91.1; by the end of the fast the average was 117.8/75.1. At a follow-up check 27 weeks after the fast the average blood pressure was 123/77.[48]

I have yet to see a case of hypertension resistant to the powerful blood-pressure-lowering effects of the fast. Even more fascinating is the observation that blood pressure does not rise back to its abnormally high level when eating is resumed. In fact, fasting, if followed by a health-supporting diet, can be a permanent cure for hypertension. Of course, if the same diet that caused the development of the high blood pressue is resumed after the fast, the problem will once again be created.

Since the blood-pressure-lowering effect of a prolonged fast continues after the fast is ended, it is not the result of the fasting-induced fluid loss, nor merely due to weight loss. Weight loss alone cannot account for the lowered blood pressure, as the results seen from fasting are significantly greater than what is generally observed from losing the same amount of weight through dieting. The lowered peripheral resistance from plaque reduction and especially the normalization of blood flow in the kidney achieved from fasting are important factors leading to the normalization of blood pressure. Fasting also results in a decrease in the size of enlarged hearts, slowing of the resting heart rate, and decreased cardiac output, all of which contribute to the permanent benefits achieved through fasting.[49,50]

Weight loss, vegetarian diets,[51] and raw foods[52] have all been shown to be effective at reducing blood pressure. Indeed, solely with such nutritional interventions, most of my patients are able to stop taking high-blood-pressure medications. Only occasionally are individuals resistant to further weight loss on an optimal diet. Sometimes the person's blood pressure does not respond to diet alone. When this is the case, I have found a therapeutic fast to be universally effective at reducing the pressure and keeping it in the desired range.

Most physicians do not offer their patients sufficiently aggressive dietary advice to enable them to improve their condition enough to stop medications. The patients who come to me have all been looking for a way to get well and off medications. The fast coupled with a nutritionally correct diet allows them to accomplish their goals.

When I discuss the futility of medical interventions and the superior results obtained with the methods discussed here with my medical colleagues or even with my physician-teachers at the medical school I attended, their typical comment is that very few people will want so restrictive a dietary approach no matter how effective. Whether this is true or not is irrelevant. We must at least offer patients the alternatives open to them and let them make the decision. It is unethical to decide for them paternalistically and withhold evidence of the effectiveness of this natural approach.

I believe many physicians would be surprised at the large percentage of patients who would choose a natural approach to recover their health rather than resort to continuous drugging and medical intervention. When individuals are educated about the side effects and risks of drugs—how they treat only the symptoms of high blood pressure without addressing the underlying cause—they routinely become very interested in the natural approach.

Patients should thoroughly understand that medications do not have a significant impact on reducing heart attacks, the leading cause of death in people with high blood pressure. In fact, because of their negative effect on lipids and glucose levels, drug treatments such as beta-blockers and diuretics may even *increase* the risk of heart attacks. Even the data from the renowned Framingham study indicate that the likelihood of death from coronary heart disease is higher during treatment with thiazide diuretics than without them.[53]

The majority of patients with high blood pressure die of heart attacks, not strokes. Medications, therefore, have been shown to have little or no effect in reducing overall cardiovascular mortality in major clinical trials.[54] Even when researchers lumped together all nine of the major hypertensive trials to achieve the statistical power of very large numbers, no significant trend was noticed in the ability of hypertensive medication to reduce the mortality or morbidity of coronary heart disease.[55]

Some of the side effects of high-blood-pressure medication are hard to ignore. They include fatigue, headache, swelling, nausea, dizziness, and many others. For example, I routinely see patients complaining of sexual dysfunction who are anxious to get off their medication.

When patients are given all the facts, including the real benefits of removing the disease rather than merely disguising its existence with drugs, they almost invariably choose the natural way to a healthy heart.

Fasting Quickly Places the High-Risk Patient at Lower Risk

Besides effectively lowering blood pressure, fasting removes and softens the cholesterol plaque that lines the blood vessels. Slowly and steadily the fast allows more blood and oxygen to circulate and thereby rejuvenate all the tissue and organs of the body.

Surgery, arthrectomy, and angioplasty, the invasive approaches to coronary artery disease, will always remain ineffective at significantly extending life. This is because these procedures address only the localized blockage. This small area of diseased blood vessel, though it may be the source of chest pain, will not necessarily be the area that causes death should a person suffer a fatal heart attack. Concentrating on a localized area of coronary artery narrowing in a body full of vessels with diffuse atherosclerotic plaque is like trying to save a patient with advanced metastatic cancer by removing one surgically accessible mass.

Understanding why a life-threatening event like a heart attack or stroke occurs lets us see why high-tech surgical methods will never significantly extend lives. Fatal or life-threatening heart attacks are typically initiated by a rupture or fissure in the atherosclerotic plaque, which leads to clot formation. A thrombus is a clot that forms within the blood vessels. The initial formation of such a clot involves the sticking together of platelets. Injury to the vessel wall releases substances, such as serotonin, that attract platelets and cause constriction or narrowing of the vessel in an attempt to stop bleeding.

Normally, clots occur to prevent bleeding from a damaged blood vessel, but a clot, or thrombus, that occurs as a result of a small fissure or ulceration in a vessel wall diseased with atherosclerosis can occlude it, leading to a heart attack or infarction (death of tissue in a specific area due to blockage of circulation). In a person with atherosclerotic heart disease, we cannot predict the spot where this fissure in the plaque and subsequent blockage will occur.

An embolus is a traveling thrombus that can occlude a small artery in the heart or brain, causing a heart attack or stroke. The main causes of strokes and heart attacks are thrombi and emboli.

While medical treatments aim at reducing symptoms and may address some discrete areas of disease, they do little or nothing to remove the underlying illness or stop its progression to an untimely death. On the other hand, fasting treats the entire body. It addresses all the biochemical abnormalities that make cardiovascular disease so dangerous. Combine this with a cholesterol-free diet before and after the fast, and patients are able to rejuvenate their cardiovascular system, safely adding years to their life.

Fasting thins the blood and prevents blood clots, or thrombi. Platelets do not clot as easily during fasting, and the ability of the red blood cells to clump together is diminished. Therefore, the fast quickly lowers an individual's risk of a heart attack.

The potential of a total fast (water only) to induce biochemical changes within the body that prevent formation of a thrombus has been well documented.[56] In one such study a fast was undertaken by 22 normal volunteers. The ability of their blood to clot and form a thrombus under fasting conditions was extensively analyzed. Fasting was discovered to lead to the reduction of blood plasma and red cell coagulation, deterioration of platelet aggregation, a rise of the oxidized hemoglobin content, and an increase in red cell resistance to peroxide hemolysis. In short, fasting lowers the risk of intravascular coagulation and thrombus formation.

Other studies have shown that after 36 hours of fasting there is a significant increase in the fibrinolytic activity of the blood. Fibrinolysis is the breakdown of clots. This activity continues for 24 hours after the fast is terminated.[57,58] Increased fibrinolysis during fasting may account for the dramatic improvement and feeling of well-being in patients suffering from thrombophlebitis (caused by clots in the blood vessels in the legs) who are fasting to treat obesity.[59]

Early in the fasting state, a significant increase in sodium and fluid excretion is predictable. This property of the fast to allow the body to excrete extra fluid has been shown to be effective as a treatment for congestive heart failure.[60] The sodium excretion and the quick loss of excessive fluid retained within the body's tissue and in the blood immediately place less stress on a diseased or weakened heart.

Fasting so effectively reduces the workload of the heart that its efficacy has even been reported in cases of intractable, severe congestive heart failure. These medical investigations began when low-salt diets and medications such as diuretics no longer sufficed to prevent the heart failure from causing fluid overload, multi-organ failure, and death, and physicians were looking for another solution.

One indication that a patient with severe chronic heart failure is entering a terminal phase is when he or she retains water, even when given diuretics and when salt intake is restricted. Several drastic measures have then been applied, including tube drainage, dialysis, and water restriction. In the search for a more successful and less harrowing program of management of these patients, fasting was tried and found to be successful in spite of failure of all other medical interventions.

In a case reported by Arthur J. Merrill, M.D., a patient who was spiraling downhill and expected to die was placed on a fast. This resulted in her recovery, enabling her to be sent home without shortness of breath or edema. Dr. Merrill states, "Had it been realized that the change would be so spectacular, a more strenuous effort would have been made to obtain accurate intake and output data with an indwelling catheter, as well as 24-hour excretions of sodium, but the patient was thought to be moribund."[61]

During the early portion of a water fast, excretion of sodium is about three times that observed with a low-salt diet. This and other biochemical parameters that favor the liquid state of the blood and lower cardiac workloads are desirable aspects of water fasting not seen with juice fasts or calorie-restricted diets. Remember, consuming only juices or any other source of calories will not give the same benefits to the cardiac patient as a total fast. Even the smallest amount of carbohydrate stops the sodium excretion.[62,63]

The fast will immediately lower or remove the risks that hang like a dagger on a thread ready to drop on disease sufferers and cut short their lives. Diets and treatments of every description flood the media, but nothing will remove these risk factors as effectively, quickly, and predictably as fasting.

A case in point is that of Robert, a 59-year-old counselor. When he came to see me he was in quite a dangerous condition, having suffered two heart attacks. A third one was obviously imminent. Robert had undergone balloon angioplasty and bypass surgery but was now suffering from recurrence of his angina (chest pain). His last angiogram showed complete blockage of two out of the three main coronary arteries and 80 percent blockage of the remaining one. He was having chest pain even as he sat in my office and described his medical history.

Robert explained that a recent stress test showed such severe cardiac insufficiency that his cardiologist had immediately stopped the test. This physician recommended repeating the bypass surgery. Robert, remembering his prior bypass experience, which almost killed him and resulted in prolonged postoperative mental confusion, decided to refuse such a risky procedure. He instead contacted Dr. Dean Ornish's office, which referred him to me.

After observing Robert for a short period of time, we began his fast. Shortly thereafter, Robert's blood pressure began to fall to a safe level and he felt better than he had in years. The biochemical changes that occur during a fast, decreasing the blood's ability to clot, lowered his risk of sudden death. His blood pressure fell to within the normal range and he enthusiastically continued his fast for a total of 24 days. His chest pain did not recur. The results of his next electrocardiogram (EKG) showed that the signs of ischemia (impaired oxygen delivery to the heart) had resolved.

No long taking any medication, Robert began to exercise—riding a bike and lifting weights—free of any pain. Today he is living a life free of any cardiac symptoms.

Another patient, Neil, underwent two balloon angioplasty procedures for recurrent angina. Within a few months after each angioplasty, his chest pain recurred, as did his severe coronary blockage, as demonstrated by repeated angiograms. He received the bad news from his physician: "You must undergo bypass surgery now as too much scar tissue has formed in the main artery of your heart and we cannot do another angioplasty." Neil refused bypass surgery and was referred to me. He underwent a 20-day fast. Soon, he was free of pain and able to play tennis and golf, and enjoy his previously active life, symptom-free. He no longer required any medication for high blood pressure or chest pain. Repeated cardiac testing (PET scans) a few months later showed that his blockage had reversed from approximately 95 percent to 60 percent. By changing his diet and fasting, he quickly reversed a dangerous cardiac condition.

For many years, Kevin had been suffering from erectile impotence and excruciating pain in his legs whenever he walked. This type of pain is called **intermittent claudication.** It is caused by blockages in the blood vessels that supply blood to the legs. The leg and hip pain began when the patient was 46, but at that time manifested itself only during significant exertions, such as long hikes. The pain slowly progressed over the years and in the last two years had become quite severe. Recently, even mild exertion such as walking 100 yards on a flat surface would generate acute pain in both legs and hips and numbness in the left foot.

Kevin consulted numerous physicians and underwent an angiogram, which documented severe atherosclerosis of the iliac arteries (major blood vessels in the leg). Immediate angioplasty of the arteries in the legs was recommended. The patient was informed there were no alternatives. Primary hypogonadism (low testosterone levels) was also diagnosed, which was thought to be the source of his impotence. He was given injections of testosterone every two weeks for the condition.

Kevin fasted for only 12 days. During the fast he continued to suffer from the above symptoms. After the fast he was first fed a small quantity of fresh fruit and vegetable juice. He progressed to melon by the end of the fourth day and was then fed raw salad and vegetables. On the fourth day of refeeding he began exercising on a stationary bike. By the seventh day of refeeding Kevin was able to walk 20 minutes without any discomfort in the legs, calves, or feet.

Upon discharge, Kevin was instructed to follow an extremely low-fat, low-protein diet, high in complex carbohydrates, vitamins, minerals, and fiber, and derived from fresh fruit, vegetables, and grains. When he returned for follow-up four weeks later, he was walking long distances without symptoms, his intermittent claudication had not returned, and he no longer required the testosterone injections as he was no longer impotent.

A fascinating aspect of fasting patients with atherosclerosis is the marked rise in cholesterol seen during the fast. Frequently patients whose cholesterol levels have gradually decreased to around 150 as a result of adopting a zero-cholesterol, plant-based diet see their cholesterol levels almost double during fasting. This large increase can occasionally continue for months after the fast is terminated. This probably reflects the breakdown of atheromas (cholesterol-laden blood vessel blockages) with release of their cholesterol contents.

Wayne, a 53-year-old man with a history of three prior angioplasties and an arthrectomy, had recurrence of his angina immediately after each of these four separate procedures. He brought his cholesterol level down from 280 to 159 by adopting a zero-cholesterol, plant-based diet, but continued to have angina while following the diet, so we began a fast about three months later. His cholesterol level on day 7 of the fast was 380; on day 14 it was 365. His angina ended on day 3 of the fast. He completed a 21-day fast and his angina has not returned. The cholesterol level normalized again to around 150 three months later.

In individuals with arterial pathways narrowed by plaque, the cholesterol levels usually increase during fasting. Young patients or those who have followed vegetarian diets for years prior to their fast, who obviously do not have fatty plaque lining their blood vessels, do not illustrate this rise in cholesterol.

A Complete Recovery Is Possible— Don't Settle for Less

It is my belief that these nutritional approaches are the medicine of the future. People who are at risk for heart attack or stroke because of high blood pressure, angina, or significant blockages in their coronary arteries can significantly extend their life span, avoid invasive medical procedures, and eliminate potentially dangerous medications for heart disease and high blood pressure. Taking advantage of today's state-of-the-art nutritional approaches makes this possible.

In my medical practice, I motivate and support patients who wish to regain control of their health. Many patients require ongoing guidance and close medical supervision during this transition. Patients quickly realize that eating a plant-based diet for better health is enjoyable and easy, not a sacrifice, and they become enthusiastic as they watch their medical problem improve and eventually resolve. I believe this type of medical care is more rewarding for the physician as well as the patient. Inevitably, more physicians will be embracing this type of care in the future.

Making significant dietary changes allows people who suffer with coronary heart disease, high cholesterol, overweight or obesity, adult diabetes, high blood pressure, and/or certain digestive and rheumatic degenerative diseases first to reduce and then to eliminate their dependence on medications and to avoid major palliative surgeries, such as heart bypass and angioplasty.

A change to a low-fat, plant-centered diet is also the most effective way to permanently lose weight and gain more energy. This, along with smoking cessation and regular exercise, reduces the risk of chronic diseases that are the leading cause of illness, death, and health-care expenditures in the United States.

Helping my patients adopt an optimal nutrition approach that will reverse, retard, or prevent disease represents the most conservative approach to the treatment of many chronic, degenerative ailments and diseases. I believe this conservative approach is also the most progressive.

6

Recovery from Diabetes Through Optimal Nutrition

One in 20 people has diabetes in this country. Diabetes, our seventh leading cause of death, is also a nutritionally related disease, one that is both preventable and reversible through nutritional methods. Like many other chronic diseases, diabetes is increasing in prevalence in the United States.

There are basically two types of diabetes: type I, or childhood-onset diabetes, and type II, or adult-onset diabetes. In type I, which generally occurs earlier in life, children incur damage to the pancreas, the organ that produces and secretes insulin, so they have an insulin deficiency. In type II, the individual still produces near-normal levels of insulin, but the body is resistant to it, so the level of blood sugar, or glucose, rises. The end result is the same in both types of the disease: the individual has a high glucose level in the blood.

Both types of diabetes accelerate the aging of our bodies. Having diabetes greatly speeds up the development of atherosclerosis, or cardiovascular disease. Diabetes also ages and destroys the kidney and other body systems. Forty thousand amputations per year are due to complications of diabetes. It is the leading cause of blindness in adults and of kidney failure.

Diabetics, regardless of the type, have abnormal blood lipids, meaning they have higher levels of triglycerides and lower levels of HDL (the "good" cholesterol) in their blood than the general population. The overproduction of triglycerides in particular is probably related to the increased flux of glucose and fatty acid substrates to the liver.[1] Unfortunately, at any given cholesterol or triglyceride level, diabetics have a much higher risk of coronary heart disease, compared to the nondiabetic population.

In both types of diabetes, the high glucose level in the blood damages the body. In conjunction with blood lipids, it inevitably causes a significant acceleration of the atherosclerotic process, hardening and narrowing the blood vessels. Atherosclerosis accounts for 80 percent of all diabetic deaths. Diabetics have more than four times as many heart attacks as nondiabetics. One third of all patients with insulin-dependent diabetes die of heart attacks before age 50.[2]

Diabetics should be made aware that they can protect themselves from becoming part of these morbid statistics. But diabetics are typically given the wrong recommendation by the professionals caring for them. You would expect that any dietary recommendations designed for diabetics would attempt to reduce the risk of a heart attack, stroke, or other cardiovascular event. Unfortunately, this is not the case. In fact, the typical dietary recommendations suggested to diabetics by their doctors and dieticians have been shown to allow the advancement of atherosclerosis in normal patients, let alone diabetics.[3,4] Both interventional studies and large epidemiologic (population-based) studies have shown conclusively that certain diets promote cardiovascular disease and diabetes, and that other nutritional practices can prevent and reverse them.

The Lifestyle Heart Trial is just one of several studies that document that the standard recommendations (utilizing a diet in which 30 percent of calories come from fat) allow the progression of heart disease even in nondiabetic patients. These recent studies were designed after it was noted in numerous population-based studies that cardiovascular deaths were virtually nonexistent in rural populations consuming vegetarian diets. In these same populations diabetes was unknown. Researchers noted that deaths from heart disease increased as populations gradually increased their consumption of animal-based foods, and that diabetes started to appear as animal foods and other rich foods were consumed.[5]

All animal foods are rich in fat and protein and deficient in fiber and the antioxidant nutrients that protect against heart disease and cancer. Many studies looking at populations consuming around 30 percent of calories from fat illustrate that such populations have a substantial amount of cardiovascular deaths, and all studies done on populations that consume less than 15 percent of calories from fat show that heart disease and diabetes are virtually nonexistent.[6]

Heart disease is the leading cause of death in diabetics. The point here is that the standard diabetic diet, which recommends 30 percent of calories from fat and usually includes salad oils, chicken, fish, and lower-fat dairy foods, is still too heavy in animal-based foods, which cause heart disease. Such a diet is risky for all people, but for the diabetic this degree of fat, cholesterol, and even protein is exceptionally hazardous. As the evidence indicates, it is a deadly diet for the diabetic.

A high-protein diet is especially risky for diabetic patients because such a diet places a significant stress on their kidneys, accelerating the progression of kidney failure.

Fat Is the Chief Enemy of the Diabetic

Fat in the diet of the diabetic not only accelerates the disease process but also interferes with the uptake of glucose by the cells, thus further raising the blood glucose level.

Experiments described in the medical literature have tested the effects of high-fat diets on insulin intolerance. In one study, healthy young medical students were fed a very high fat diet containing egg yolks, heavy cream, and butter, and within two days all of the students had blood sugar levels high enough to be labeled diabetic.[7] Complex carbohydrates have been shown to have the opposite effect.[8]

Fat in the food we eat prevents the proper utilization of insulin, and more insulin is needed to process the glucose when fats are

129

included in the meal. Additionally, the fat on one's body makes the cells resistant to insulin, and the pancreas must produce more insulin to compensate. This is due not only to the additional insulin demanded by the extra body mass of fat cells, but also to the fact that the fat in and around normal tissue, like muscle and internal organs, interferes with insulin uptake into these tissues. The major contributors to fat in the American diet are animal-source foods such as meat, fowl, fish, and dairy products, as well as cooking or salad oils.

Insulin Is the Accomplice in Crime

After World War I, when insulin was first discovered, the medical profession thought diabetes would be totally curable as a medical problem. Diabetes was believed to be due to insulin deficiency, and everyone thought that since insulin would now be given to patients there would be no more problems. It seemed this way for a few years, but terrible things started happening to patients with diabetes who were given insulin to control their blood sugar levels. They developed eye disease, kidney disease, and, most important, accelerating atherosclerosis leading to blood vessel disease and early heart attacks. Their problems were worse than ever.

Decades later, when the insulin assay became available and doctors were able to measure insulin levels in their patients' bloodstreams, they found most interesting results: the insulin levels of type I (childhood-onset) diabetics were indeed low, but the levels in type II (adult-onset) diabetics were not only not low, but also were higher than those of people without diabetes.

It became clear that type II diabetics is a disease of insulin resistance, not insulin deficiency. Type II diabetics produce plenty of insulin, but for some reason still not enough to drive the glucose from the bloodstream into the cells.

If we measured the insulin level in prediabetic people (those who will become diabetic years later), we would find insulin levels much higher than normal. These persons consume excesses of fat, sugar, protein, and refined or processed foods and have excess fat on their bodies; as a result their pancreas must secrete increased amounts of insulin to overcome the insulin-blocking effects of their fat cells and the fat they ingest.

All overweight individuals, whether diabetic or not, have abnormally high levels of circulating insulin. In fact, being overweight can force one's body to manufacture up to four to five times as much insulin as a normal person. Many obese individuals eventually become diabetic. About 85 percent of adult diabetics are significantly overweight.

Some of the obese may never become diabetic because their pancreatic reserve may enable them to continue to produce this excessive amount of insulin for years. Even if they never become diabetic, however, the high levels of insulin contribute to their cardiovascular risk by increasing the process of atherosclerosis. Insulin increases the rate at which cholesterol-laden plaque builds up on arterial walls. The abnormally high levels of insulin produced by all overweight individuals, diabetic or not, is an independent risk factor for early cardiac death.

After years of this unusual stress, the pancreas starts to tire out and eventually can secrete only normal amounts of insulin in response to the high demand by the body. This occurs because we all lose some beta cell function as we age (beta cells are the cells in the pancreas that secrete insulin) and excessive demand causes an acceleration of this process. Now, 8 to 20 years later, the pancreas finally says "enough is enough" and slowly stops producing high levels of insulin. At this point the glucose level in the blood begins to rise, and the person may notice the first signs that something is wrong, such as increased urination. Diabetes is then diagnosed. These are the major factors causing adult-onset diabetes.

The seeds of diabetes are planted by high insulin levels many years before a person becomes a diabetic. This is when the damaging effects of the elevated insulin begin to hurt the body, long before the disease is diagnosed. When a person first develops the signs and symptoms of type II (adult-onset) diabetes, the problem has existed for a long time. Typically the body has been battling with excessive insulin requirements and the pancreas has been overworked to exhaustion for more than ten years before the level of glucose rises in the bloodstream. If we could have tested insulin levels of an individual every year for ten years before diagnosis, we would have found high and rising insulin levels.

When the diagnosis of diabetes is first made, the individual may already have other related medical complications. In fact, many of these patients actually come to physicians because of these complications, such as a heart attack, and then the physician notices this person's glucose is a little high. But such individuals so often never knew they had diabetes until a medical complication of diabetes made them come to the doctor. This is because excess insulin is very damaging to the body—especially to the circulation, including the large blood vessels as well as the small ones in the eyes and kidneys. All those years of excessive insulin secretion take their toll, resulting in extensive damage to the body.

The tendency of the pancreas eventually to lose the ability to produce such excessive amounts of insulin may be influenced by genetics. Thirty to 40 years ago the Pima and Tohono O'odham Indian tribes of the American Southwest ate cactus, roots, berries, beans, corn, and greens. Diabetes was unknown in their ancestry. Eventually these Native American tribes adopted the standard American diet. As a result, more than half of these Indians presently become diabetic by the age of 35, although before 1945 diabetes was unknown in this population.[9]

Multiple other studies show similar patterns when societies adopt modern diets.[10,11] Therefore, the inherited tendency to develop diabetes may be there, but that does not mean we have to stress our bodies so much that this inherited weakness becomes evident.

When Earl Ray, a Pima Indian who lives near Phoenix, switched back to a more traditional Native American diet of mesquite meal, beans, and cactus fruit, his weight dropped from 239 pounds to less than 150 pounds and his severe diabetes was controlled without medication.

So fat and glucose are not the only villains. The high levels of insulin present in diabetics also promote hardening of the blood vessels and aging of the body. Findings from numerous studies have shown that insulin blocks cholesterol removal, stimulates the formation of atherosclerotic plaques, and contributes to the delivery of cholesterol to the cells. Insulin also promotes other damage such as smooth muscle and connective tissue proliferation.[12, 13] This leads to even more blood vessel stiffness and damage, because the muscular wall of the blood vessel becomes thicker and less elastic as the interior lining becomes laden with atherosclerotic plaque, thus increasing the diabetic's risk of stroke and heart attack.

So insulin is a great villain. In fact, if you want to have your blood taken for just one blood test that will be the best indicator of your risk for heart attack in the next ten years, get a serum insulin level, not a serum cholesterol.

Insulin obviously has some essential functions in the body. It allows the uptake of glucose by the cells, thus giving our cells energy, but it also drives the growth of fat and helps us store our excess nutrients in the form of body fat. Extra insulin also can slow down one's metabolic rate as it efficiently aids the process of packing away more fat on the body. So the heavier one becomes, the more insulin the body needs to make, and the more insulin the body produces (or is given), the fatter—and the more diabetic, or insulin-resistant—one becomes.

So it is absolutely essential that type II diabetics maintain a slim physique. Sometimes type II diabetics who think they are not overweight can loose ten pounds of fat they didn't think they had and, like magic, their glucose levels normalize.

Standard Recommendations for Diabetes

Now that you understand the mechanism that leads to the development of adult-onset, or type II, diabetes, let's look at the current methods for treating diabetes. The American Diabetic Association recommends restricting fat intake to 30 percent of

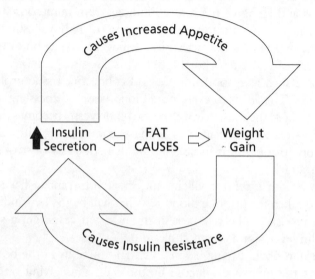

Causes Increased Appetite

Insulin Secretion ⇐ FAT CAUSES ⇒ Weight Gain

Causes Insulin Resistance

calories from fat. Patients follow an exchange diet to keep daily calories constant. A low-protein diet is sometimes recommended only after the kidneys show damage.

The 30-percent-of-calories-from-fat recommendation is the same number used by the American Heart Association and other governmental authorities in this country. When this diet fails to adequately control blood sugar levels, oral medication is used to stimulate the pancreas to produce more insulin. When this fails, insulin injections are used to attempt to bring glucose levels near normal. When this fails, both insulin and oral medication are used.

The Remedy Is Worse Than the Disease

The administration of insulin and oral medications attempts to address only one aspect of the problem—the increased blood sugar levels. Because insulin increases one's appetite and increases glucose uptake by the cells, the diabetic patient becomes more diabetic and eventually requires more insulin, and so on. Increased insulin is responsible for increased death from heart attacks. Giving a type II diabetic insulin is like giving an alcoholic more alcohol.

Hypoglycemic pills (the oral diabetes medication) are not as bad as insulin; however, they too have been shown to increase the risk of dying from heart disease 2.5 times more than that of diabetics treated by diet alone. They can cause dangerous side effects such as jaundice, anemia, skin rashes, and even, though rarely, death.[14] But the main problem is that the blood-sugar-lowering effect of these medications is achieved mainly through stimulating the pancreatic islet cells to produce more insulin. Attempting to stimulate the weakened pancreas eventually takes its toll, aggravating the loss of beta cell function. Thus, again, the person is likely to become more diabetic. The oral medications also increase glucose and fatty acid uptake in skeletal muscles and fat cells, helping the person gain weight more easily and become more diabetic.[15,16]

Both insulin and oral hypoglycemic agents can also cause potentially life-threatening episodes of hypoglycemia, or low blood sugar. Both medications, when compared to diet control, accelerate the aging of the diabetic, accelerate the complications of the disease, and aid in the early death of the diabetic.

Today's typical treatment combined with the usual American Diabetic Association diet is a proven dangerous approach. The ADA-recommended diet has been shown to promote heart disease in patients who do not have diabetes. Therefore, in the diabetic it is an extremely foolish practice. Feeding a diabetic a high-fat diet including multiple daily servings of chicken, meat, fish, and dairy products will greatly accelerate his or her death. Then, when we combine this with the typical treatments offered by most physicians, it is no wonder diabetics suffer from multiple medical complications and die an unnecessarily early death. I can only view today's treatment of diabetic patients as malpractice, yet it is the standard of care. If they are not given this basic information, we are depriving them of their opportunity for wellness and normal life spans.

A Plant-Based Diet Is an Effective Approach to Treating Diabetes

When Elizabeth first came to me she weighed 222 pounds, she was taking 115 units of insulin daily, and her fasting blood sugar levels were between 250 and 300. Her prior physician was concerned that her diabetes was still so poorly controlled on increasing doses of insulin. He did not know what more he could do and suggested adding an oral hypoglycemic medication to the high dose of insulin to see if the sugar levels could be better controlled.

Instead, Elizabeth saw me and we started a more effective approach. I cut her insulin back to a total of 70 units daily as she began following my dietary suggestions. She phoned two days later to report that her blood sugar levels were running between 130 and 152, so we cut the insulin back to 40 units per day. She returned for a follow-up visit a few days later, one week after her initial appointment, and was doing so well that she had stopped her insulin completely the day before. Her sugars were now running below 150 and she had lost 7 pounds during that first week. She went from using 115 units of insulin a day while her diabetes was under poor control to requiring no insulin at all, and this took place in merely one week's time. She is continuing to lose weight.

The diet plan to reverse diabetes and enable patients to eliminate their dependence on drugs is one derived from vegetables, fruits, grains, and legumes. Refined and overly processed foods, convenience foods, and foods that are high in refined carbohydrates, salt, and other additives should all be avoided for good health. The diabetic, who is even more sensitive to the harmful effects of the American diet, should take care to consume a natural plant-based diet with an abundance of raw vegetables in the form of large salads every day. It is essential that the diabetic avoid concentrated vegetable oils including margarine, olive oil, corn oil, and other fats. Nuts, olives and avocados are also best left out of the diet due to their fat content.

A large green salad, eaten daily, is the only food that has shown a significant correlation with longer life in scientific studies.[17,18] Guar and other water-soluble fibers in beans, oats, barley, and fruit are also important, and are present in large quantities in a plant-based diet. No sweets except for fresh fruit should be eaten. Fruit juices and dried fruit should also be limited or avoided.

Weight loss in even the slightly overweight diabetic is essential, so regular exercise is an important part of the prescription. Both aerobic and weight training or Nautilus-type exercise should be done on a regular basis to keep a very high muscle-to-fat ratio in the body. The goal is to make the body "lean and mean."

When following the above recommendations, patients lose weight and their blood sugar levels drop immediately. Additionally, the low protein content of this diet protects the kidneys.

This program is so effective that I have developed the position that a diabetic patient who is not a strict vegetarian is either ill-informed or foolish. Doctors who know this information are irresponsible if they do not explain it to their patients.

Nutritional Supplements Are Not the Answer

Many nutrients are often touted as effective remedies for the diabetic. Chromium, for example, has been shown to improve glycemic control in diabetics who are chromium deficient. Supplementation with vitamin E has also been shown to have a favorable effect on blood sugar control in diabetics.[19] Vitamin C supplementation to 1,000 mg per day has been shown to retard the damaging effects of glucose on body proteins, thus lessening the damage from the high glucose levels in diabetes and retarding the aging process.[20]

The point to remember is that every nutrient that has been shown to have a favorable effect on glucose control is present in abundance in fresh fruits and vegetables and deficient in processed foods, dairy foods, and animal foods. When we consume a diet of primarily raw and conservatively cooked plant foods, we consume very high levels of these nutrients, plus nutritional factors that have not yet been discovered or isolated and that are essential for optimal health. More than six hundred antioxidants have been identified so far, many of which work synergistically (strengthening the protective effects of the other nutrients they accompany) with other compounds to produce observed effects, such as LDL oxidation. Obviously, we can get adequate amounts of all these beneficial nutrients only by eating an abundance of unprocessed natural foods (many of the protective nutrients are lost in processing). Merely adding supplements to an inadequate diet will never suffice.

If you are on the optimal diet already, will taking extra amounts of vitamins E and C and chromium be important? The answer is probably not. A natural plant-based diet already provides more than 1,000 mg of vitamin C, for example. Only time and further research will tell if the diabetic will benefit further from supplementation once he or she is eating optimally. If you are on the standard American diet or a diet recommended by the typical health professional, similar to the suggestions of the American Diabetic Association (a diet that I consider dangerous for diabetics), then it would make sense to supplement your diet with other nutrients such as superoxide dismutase complex, rutin, bioflavonoids, and carotenoids, since those diets are significantly lacking in essential protective nutrients, especially antioxidants.

Fasting Can Aid in Recovery from Diabetes

Fasting can play an important part in the recovery from adult-onset diabetes. In fact, early in this century, many years before insulin was ever used to treat diabetics, fasting was used as an important therapeutic modality to prolong life in diabetic patients.[21] It was reported at that time that even in severe cases of adult diabetes, the signs and symptoms of the disease resolve with fasting. Glycosuria and acidosis resolved with recovery occurring even in the weak and emaciated patients.

In these early studies on fasting done at the Hospital of the Rockefeller Institute for Medical Research in New York, the physicians employing this therapy noted that "fasting has not appeared harmful even in these few cases where it has not been successful." Even in these early investigations the importance of keeping the patient permanently "below weight" after the fast and the importance of restricting the quantity of fat in the diet to maintain the benefit gained from the fast were repeatedly emphasized. The authors stated, "Anyone can readily convince himself that, in a suitably severe diabetic who is symptom-free for days or weeks (after a fast) and on a fixed diet, the addition of some quantity of butter or olive oil to the diet will bring back the glycosuria, ketonuria and other symptoms immediately or within a short time."

Unfortunately, now that physicians are able to control these symptoms with drugs, these pearls of knowledge gleaned by researchers from the days when no drugs were available are largely ignored.

More recent studies reporting on the fasting of diabetic patients have likewise shown excellent results,[22,23,24] and confirm the changes I see with my patients. They concluded that, following a prolonged fast, the diabetic patient shows a substantial improvement in insulin function independent of the degree of weight loss, and restoration of pancreatic function can occur that does not occur with weight loss alone. Complete remission of diabetes was reported in many patients.

Fasting should not be used early in the treatment, but rather after many months on the diabetic reversal diet, when the person has lost most of the excessive weight. At this point an extended fast can remove the last bit of difficult-to-lose weight and, more important, can give the pancreas a chance to rest so it can reset its sensitivity to glucose and recover its normal function. The fast is useful especially when the person is doing fairly well, but still has mildly elevated fasting glucose levels after following the optimal diet and having restored normal or near normal weight.

If the fast is used correctly in the type II diabetic (type I diabetics should not fast), it increases beta cell sensitivity to glucose, which can restore integrity to the pancreas and allow it to reestablish its sensitivity to glucose. This is an important therapeutic modality to bring diabetics whose sugar levels are relatively well controlled with optimal diet to the point where, after a fast is completed, the blood sugars remain entirely within the normal range while the same diet is continued.

Using fasting in a later phase of the treatment program results in restoration of pancreatic function so that patients regain normal blood sugar levels and, in many cases, have no further findings indicative of diabetes. Fasting too early in the treatment program may temporarily slow the metabolic rate, actually making further weight loss more difficult, especially if the individual is not lean after the fast.

When Bill first came to see me, he had already suffered from one heart attack. He was taking an oral hypoglycemic medication for his diabetes, as well as other drugs. I stopped his oral diabetic medication at the first visit, and he began my recommended diet for diabetes. When Bill returned two weeks later his blood sugar levels were around 140, much better than they had been on the medication, with his previous diet. His blood pressure remained high, however (180/95 while taking the Tenormin, a blood-pressure-lowering medication), and we decided to begin a fast rather than add further medication at this time. When he arrived a week later to begin his fast, he already had lost about 10 pounds since I had first seen him about three weeks earlier. All medications were stopped and he fasted 20 days. When Bill completed his fast, he had lost 20 more pounds, and not only did his blood pressure remain around 110/70 without medication, but also his fasting glucose levels stayed under 120, within the normal range.

Occasionally, a diabetic patient who is significantly overweight may need to eat correctly, exercise appropriately, fast, continue to eat correctly for a few months, and fast again. In this manner the overweight diabetic grows lean and strong. By combining exercise and extremely low fat, high-fiber, plant diets with fasting, the patient builds a new body. Both the patient and I develop excitement at the new, lean, trim, muscular body that eventually reveals itself from under the old cloak of fat. Like training for and competing in the Olympic Games, these patients reach their own sustained triumph as they recover and maintain their health.

The combination of fasting, which places the least demand possible on the patient's overworked pancreas, with the lower insulin demands of the new diet gives the pancreas its well-earned rest and enables the body to accomplish internal house-cleaning and to repair cells damaged by years of diabetes. Importantly, since all diabetics have significant blood vessel disease with hardening of the arteries diffusely throughout their vessels, the fast is able to address the damage already done. Like no other therapeutic modality, fasting removes the risk of a cardiovascular accident or other complication that was practically inevitable without this intervention.

Before insulin was discovered earlier in this century, many patients with diabetes were treated in the manner described—by very low fat diets and fasting. The medical profession abandoned the practice after insulin was discovered because physicians of the time thought diabetes was licked and that no one should have to deprive him- or herself of food in order to get well. Insulin gave diabetics the freedom to continue to be fat, to continue to abuse their bodies, and to continue to allow their body to age and weaken from the effects of diabetes without having the immediate symptoms of dry mouth, frequent urination, and weakness. But now we know better.

So we must get diabetics off their treatments. If the sugars are not adequately controlled with diet alone, then fasting must be used. If the diabetic is motivated and truly wants the best opportunity for a long healthy life, we should not use medication at all in type II diabetes; instead, we should utilize aggressive nutritional intervention with fasting, the most effective treatment for these patients.

My results, obtained from diabetics adopting this natural

approach, show that over 95 percent of type II diabetics can come off medications with much better blood sugar control than they had on insulin or oral medication. With the dietary modifications alone, type I, or childhood-onset, diabetics are able to reduce their insulin requirements by almost half. But more important, they can improve their overall health, retard the destruction of their bodies, and significantly reduce complications and the risk of early cardiac death.

All physicians should inform their patients about the optimal recommendations to maximize their life span and minimize their risk of suffering from disease complications. Then at least the patient can make an educated and informed choice. If this prescription is followed, heart attacks and strokes will become rare. Diabetes will diminish in incidence and practically disappear from our society.

We can help ourselves, our friends, and our children adopt eating habits they can live with so that they can be free of the fear of heart disease, stroke, diabetes, and many other serious illnesses. Passing on to you this valuable information gives you the power to free yourself from medical treatments, to control your own life, and to choose your own health destiny.

NOTE: No patient on medication should make dietary changes without the assistance of a physician, as medication adjustment will be necessary to prevent excessive lowering of the blood sugar level, or hypoglycemia.

7 | Autoimmune Disease: A Superior Approach

A patient's wife wrote, "My husband has been seeking medical help for the past two and a half years for rheumatoid arthritis. He was going for blood tests every two to six weeks. He was using Azulfidine, Prednisone and Methotrexate along with other prescribed drugs. He was about to begin gold shots when he changed physicians. Thank God he did! He would not die from the arthritis, but from the side effects of the treatments. After three months Dr. Fuhrman has my husband off all drugs." The patient added, "Six months ago I prayed I would die, now I'm ready to live again."
                                                    —Mr. and Mrs. Priatt

From the Priatts' unsolicited remarks one can see why I am so enthusiastic about the treatment of autoimmune diseases with diet and fasting. I have consistently watched my patients recover from what they have been told are incurable illnesses.

There are more than a hundred clinical syndromes labeled as autoimmune disease. Those discussed in this chapter are serious medical illnesses. They cause pain, suffering, and early death. Drugs, the present-day treatment, have extremely serious side effects. As a matter of fact, the toxic effects of the drugs can be worse than the diseases themselves. It is not uncommon that patients are unable to tolerate the medications prescribed by their physicians.

The good news is that in the majority of cases these diseases respond predictably to fasting and plant-based diets. To get optimal results, these diets must be modified for the particular needs of each patient.

It is also predictable that in spite of well-conducted scientific investigations and the clinical experience of many physicians, this effective nutritional treatment of autoimmune disease is generally ignored. This is unfortunate, because optimal nutrition alone can prevent the suffering of millions.

It is important to note that the fact that a particular autoimmune disease is not discussed in this chapter does not mean it will not be helped or alleviated by this approach. Autoimmune illnesses that I will not discuss, but that *do* typically respond to this type of treatment include Hashimoto's thyroiditis, nephritis, Sjögren's syndrome, connective tissue disorders, and others. Even some diseases not generally classified as autoimmune actually improve with this approach because they have mechanisms the same as or similar to those outlined in this chapter. These include asthma, allergic disorders such as rhinitis, and various dermatologic disorders such as eczema, urticaria, and dermatitis herpetiformis.

What Is Autoimmune Disease?

The body's defense system against foreign invaders is called the **immune system.** This finely tuned system is constantly adjusting itself with checks and controls in an attempt to remove substances foreign or toxic to it.

Sometimes the body's internal defenses make a mistake; they see an enemy where in reality there is none, or they respond uncontrollably to a minor insult. The term **autoimmune disease** was coined to reflect the body's misinterpretations.

Normally, the intricate activities of the immune system effectively distinguish between the body's own cells and cellular debris and foreign infiltrators. In autoimmune disorders this recognition breaks down, and the body's own cells are attacked. In effect, the body loses its ability to tell the difference between foreign substances and itself. When this occurs, the immune system generates antibodies against its own tissues, and may begin to attack, inflame, and destroy itself.

The miscommunication of the body's internal defense structure happens for two reasons: one, because the cells may have been altered in some way that makes them appear foreign to immune recognition, and two, because some aspect controlling immune activity has gone awry.

All cells have protein and lipid projections on their outer walls that serve as identifying markers to the immune system. Antibodies are designed so that they can bind with a cell's outer surface projections, much the way a key fits into a lock. Thus the antibodies can attach themselves to the cell and recognize whether the cell looks normal or not. If through this contact with the surface of the cell the immune markers tag the cell as abnormal, other, larger components of the immune system will be attracted to destroy the so-labeled body cell.

As we place disease-causing stressors on our body throughout our lives, our cells can become biochemically weak and congested with self-generated wastes. Eventually, as waste accumulates within the cell, it overtaxes the cell's detoxifying ability. More and more waste is then forced into the cellular wall, which will eventually mark the cell as aged and abnormal to immune surveillance. The immune system will at this point begin its job of attacking this cell in an attempt to remove it. Therefore, in many autoimmune illnesses, cellular detoxification via nutritional management and fasting is essential for achieving improvement or recovery because these measures allow the cells to reduce their load of metabolic wastes and therefore appear normal again to immune surveillance.

In multiple sclerosis, for example, part of the myelin sheath that protects nerves is attacked and destroyed. For some reason these cells look abnormal to the immune system. In hemolytic anemia red blood cells are attacked and destroyed, and in Graves' disease thyroid cells are attacked and stimulated, causing excessive secretion of thyroid hormone.

In rheumatoid arthritis, the immune system attacks and inflames the joints. In psoriasis, the attack is directed against the skin, and in inflammatory bowel disease (ulcerative colitis and Crohn's) the digestive tract becomes the site of the immune hyperactivity. Systemic lupus erythematosus (SLE) is a chronic inflammatory disease that can affect various parts of the body, especially the skin, joints, blood, and kidneys.

Besides recognizing cellular deviance, the immune system can cause damage for other reasons, especially from the formation and accumulation of immune complexes in our tissues.

In order to protect us, our immune system first has to identify the object it wants to attack. The antibodies attach themselves to foreign substances, debris, and dead or abnormal cells. They identify this interior pollution so that the other part of the immune system, the immune cells, can be attracted to the area and gobble up or destroy the offending substance. When an antibody attaches itself to an offending substance, called the antigen, an antigen–antibody complex is formed.

These complexes are present in the blood in increased quantities in individuals with autoimmune illnesses. When these complexes are not effectively cleared from the bloodstream, they can become lodged in various tissues, where they cause inflammation, much like a sliver of wood does when it is caught under the skin.

In rheumatoid arthritis, for example, these complexes are deposited in the joints, and redness, swelling, stiffness, and pain develop, followed by destruction of the joint as the inflammation continues. The amount of immune complexes deposited in the joints corresponds to the severity of the arthritic symptoms.[1]

Autoimmune Disease Equals
Digestive Dysfunction

The number one source of this excessive immune complex formation is **digestive tract malfunction,** often called "the leaky gut syndrome."

It has been shown in scientific studies that many people with rheumatoid arthritis and other autoimmune diseases have increased intestinal tract permeability.[2,3] Because of genetic or other insults to the digestive system earlier in life, autoimmune disease sufferers have an abnormality of the digestive tract that allows incompletely digested foodstuffs to pass through the intestinal lining and enter the bloodstream.

Proteins in foods are the chief culprits that can excite an abnormal immune response. A protein is typically made up of thousands of amino acids linked together. The digestive enzymes cleave the bonds between the amino acids during digestion, allowing the individual amino acids to pass through the wall of the digestive tract. When isolated amino acids enter the bloodstream, they do not excite an (abnormal) immune response. During the process of digesting the protein, however, if a piece of partially broken-down protein, known as a peptide, is able to pass through the digestive tract wall by mistake, this peptide can and will excite the immune system to react against it.

The peptide, containing perhaps a hundred amino acids, is now recognized not as a nutrient like an individiual amino acid, but rather as a foreign substance that needs to be attacked and removed. Thus, the immune system produces an antibody to this antigen, and an antigen–antibody complex is formed.

It is clear that the intestinal tract is a critical interface between the external world and our tightly regulated inner environment. When this critical line of defense is disrupted, enzymes, bacteria-elaborated toxins, immunostimulating peptides, and other unwanted substances may escape the mucosal defenses of the digestive tract and enter the bloodstream. The result is circulating immune complexes that can induce autoimmune disease, joint inflammation, and pain.

Meat and Other Animal Foods Are Implicated in Autoimmune Illnesses

There is evidence that when peptides from animal proteins are absorbed, they not only can lead to the formation of antibodies against them, but also can cross-react against human proteins in the body. This may be because animal meats have amino acid sequences that are similar to those found in human tissue. Plant proteins are less likely to cause this reaction, even if their peptides pass into the bloodstream, because they bear little resemblance to human proteins.

When the immune system views the animal peptides in the bloodstream and attempts to attack and destroy them, the antibodies created can continue to attack other body tissues later. Because amino acid sequences in human body proteins are similar to those of the animal peptides, these antibodies can attach to and cause a reaction to one's own tissues.

Excess protein in the diet creates a significant risk for the development of autoimmune disease because, by nature, we are designed like the other large primates to consume comparatively low amounts of protein.

When we eat an animal-food-based diet with servings of high-protein animal foods at each meal, our capacity to digest this food efficiently is strained. Unlike the true carnivorous animals, which can secrete large quantities of acids in their digestive tracts and huge amounts of protein-cleaving enzymes to aid in the digestive process, the human animal cannot. Because we cannot efficiently dissolve these proteins, more incompletely digested peptides are apt to be absorbed. In addition, our intestines allow more bacteria species to overgrow when this environment is rich with animal-food-derived peptides. This results in the absorption of toxic bacterial by-products, which can create an inflammatory environment. So the overgrowth of various bacterial species thriving in the gut of the average American contributes to immune dysfunction.

The excess of fat in the diet from either animal fats or excessive vegetable oil can impede the ability of the body quickly to clear immune complexes from the bloodstream. Excess fat hinders immune function.[4] The immune complexes created by gut leakage are not adequately removed because their removal is impeded by fat consumption. The complexes then circulate for long periods and eventually deposit themselves in our tissues. This impairment of the immune system by fats is one reason the present-day Western diet is associated with such a high rate of cancer and autoimmune disease.

So rheumatoid arthritis, the most common of the autoimmune-type illnesses, is not merely a joint disease. It is a problem of the entire body, starting with the digestive tract. Joint pain is one of the most common autoimmune symptoms simply because the joints are particularly vulnerable to immune insults.

The joints receive nutrients and remove wastes through the joint fluid. Joint areas are extremely sensitive to decreased oxygenation because they have a marginal blood supply to begin with. Instead of being directly fed by blood vessels, the joints must receive their oxygenation via the joint fluid. When a fatty meal is consumed, the blood thickens and red blood cells stick together, which reduces the oxygenation of all tissues. This has a significant effect on the oxygenation of joint tissues, increasing the sensitivity of joints to inflammation and immune system damage. Decreased oxygenation alone can cause inflammation.

Even young people who have not yet narrowed the major blood vessels supplying the heart and major organs may have impairment of circulation to the microscopic vasculature around the joints. Decreased oxygen causes inflammation, which attracts antigen–antibody complexes to be deposited. Decreased oxygenation also can prevent repair of the microscopic fractures that occur in the joint area from normal activity. Additionally, because the area around the joint capsule is poorly supplied with blood, it is less effective at removing metabolic wastes and toxins that may accumulate in this area.

When the marginal blood supply to a joint is further compromised by narrowing of the small blood vessels from atherosclerotic plaque or by the sludging of blood (stickiness of the red blood cells) that occurs after a fatty meal, the joint tissues become more prone to arthritic damage. This is one reason why the joints are a common site for the manifestation of autoimmune disease.

Drug Treatment of Autoimmune Disease Poses Serious Risks

Autoimmune diseases destroy the body by similar mechanisms, and they are treated by similar drugs. When we look at the use of drugs to treat rheumatologic or autoimmune illnesses, we see serious side effects as well as damaging and dangerous long-term effects. What follows is only a partial list of drug-related side effects.

NSAIDs (nonsteroidal anti-inflammatory drugs) such as salicylates (aspirin and related compounds) have retained their preeminent position in the treatment of rheumatic disease for almost a hundred years. Motrin, Naprosyn, Feldene, and Ansaid are newer NSAIDs. Drugs in this category are generally considered the safest of the medications used for autoimmune illnesses. They are well known for the side effects of irritation of the stomach lining, ulcer disease, and gastrointestinal bleeding. They can also cause diarrhea, nausea, constipation, dry mouth, headache, dizziness, ringing in the ears, liver or kidney disease, nervousness, swelling, and septic meningitis.[5]

Several studies have shown that NSAIDs actually accelerate the progression of arthritis by further damaging the mucosal lining of the digestive tract.[6] This causes more intestinal permeability and more passage of incompletely digested food and bacterial toxins that worsen the underlying autoimmune disease.

Steroids, such as prednisone, are effective medications for autoimmune illnesses because they quickly suppress the inflammatory response. Side effects include electrolyte disturbances, diabetes, increased susceptibility to infection including tuberculosis, peptic ulcers (which may bleed or perforate), osteoporosis, cataracts, obesity, moon face (the face becomes swollen and round), buffalo hump (characterized by a lump of fatty tissue that grows in the back between the shoulder blades), acne, nervousness, insomnia, depression, schizophrenia, and suicide.

Withdrawal of prednisone can cause muscle and joint pain, as well as weakness. These symptoms from the drug may be extremely difficult to distinguish from the disease (such as rheumatoid arthritis) itself.[7]

Chemotherapeutic agents (also used to treat cancer and leukemia) such as methotrexate and Imuran can be effective in controlling symptoms but have dangerous long-term effects such as causing cancer. They work by attacking the immune system, which also is the basis of their toxic side effects. Other side effects include bone marrow destruction, platelet destruction with massive bleeding, bleeding from the digestive tract, death due to gastrointestinal perforation, hair loss, liver and kidney impairment, potentially fatal infections, and both solid tumor cancers and leukemia.[8,9]

Gold, typically used for rheumatoid arthritis, can cause intestinal bleeding, gold lung, severe skin rashes, life-threatening bone marrow disease (including severe anemia), decreased platelets, kidney and liver damage, and hair loss.[10] The use of gold compounds has been shown to be among the most common drug-induced causes of death.[11]

Plaquenil, most often used for lupus or arthritis, can cause the following: irreversible visual loss from retinal damage, anxiety, nightmares, psychosis, hair loss, hearing loss, and skin eruptions such as psoriasis.[12]

Thousands of patients die each year or become seriously ill from the side effects of the above medications. Obviously, it makes sense to try a safe, conservative approach to getting well before spending a lifetime on these toxic, dangerous drugs.

Diet Is Critical in Rheumatoid Arthritis

Arthritis sufferers spend more than $1 billion annually on drug treatment. One million new cases are diagnosed every year, and the number is growing. Five percent of America's elderly population suffer from this disease. It is called the "nation's primary crippler."[13] Recent studies have refuted the previously held notion that rheumatoid arthritis has a favorable outcome. Patients experience progressive decline in joint mobility and generally get steadily worse in spite of today's toxic treatments. Such patients generally have a four- to ten-year decrease in life expectancy.

More significantly, the prognosis is very poor for persons who have progressed to multiple joint involvement. The five-year survival rate for severely arthritic individuals with multiple joint involvement is about 45 percent.[14] Similar low survival rates are observed in patients with other very serious illnesses, such as Hodgkin's disease and three-vessel coronary artery disease.

Traditionally, when less toxic medications are unable to control symptoms or when the side effects became intolerable, the physician will consider using more powerful and more toxic chemotherapeutic agents, which have even more dangerous side effects, including cancer.

In recent years, rheumatologists have been starting patients on the more toxic chemotherapeutic agents earlier, or even as a primary approach, in a purely theoretical attempt to slow down the progression of the disease. This practice is prevalent even though there is little evidence to prove that it holds long-term benefit for the patient. Although medications can reduce inflammation and pain, the evidence collected so far indicates these drugs have little or no effect on long-term outcome.[15,16]

Another recent study of arthritis patients reported that after 20 years of treatments with the typical drugs including prednisone, methotrexate, penicillamine, and oral gold, half the patients were either dead or disabled.[17] The idea that drugs induce remissions was described as "fallacious." The unfortunate reality is that drug therapy often contributes to the suffering and early death of the arthritis patient.

How can anyone argue that safe and potentially curative modalities such as fasting and natural diet should not be tried first? In spite of numerous and repeated proclamations by the American Arthritis Association and rheumatologists to the contrary, rheumatoid arthritis is preventable and reversible. Fasting and vegetarian diet have proven to be the only effective way to achieve consistent remission in such patients.

The Arthritis Foundation boldly declares in their literature that there is no special diet for arthritis, and that food has nothing to do with causing it. Fortunately, there is solid evidence to refute this ill-informed and irresponsible opinion.

First there is the epidemiologic evidence. In populations that consume natural diets of mostly unprocessed fruits, vegetables, and grains, autoimmune diseases are almost nonexistent. Rheumatoid arthritis, ankylosing spondylitis, psoriasis, and psoriatic arthritis are exceptionally rare in China, Indonesia, and Africa, where the populations consume vegetarian or near-vegetarian diets.[18,19] The same is found with lupus. Whereas African blacks rarely develop this disease, it has a high prevalence in the United States, especially among black women.[20]

This cannot be because of heredity or racial differences. When people migrate from China, Indonesia, Japan, and Africa to the United States and begin to consume a rich western diet, arthritis and other autoimmune diseases become common.

When these diseases do crop up in such populations, they are not severe. The people generally have a milder form of the disease, without the joint deformities and the significant reduction of life span that we see in this country.[21]

So will placing people with rheumatoid arthritis on natural-food, plant-based diets help our autoimmune-disease-ridden population? The results of studies done on dairy-free, plant-based diets have been impressive. In a study at Wayne University Medical School, fat-free diets were fed to volunteers, and resulted in complete remission of arthritis in the majority of participants. All the participants relapsed when either vegetable oils or animal food was reintroduced into their diets. The investigators concluded that the high-fat, high-protein American diet causes rheumatoid arthritis.[22]

Fasting Can Be Effective in Treating Autoimmune Illnesses

Fasting is a remarkable anti-inflammatory intervention, more powerful than the strongest and most toxic drugs at reducing inflammation. It is a crucial management tool for the person suffering from autoimmunal disease, and, when combined with appropriate dietary modifications, can induce a remission of symptoms.

A supervised fast is the most effective way the individual with rheumatoid arthritis can quickly eliminate pain and stop the degeneration of the body and joints caused by the attack of the immune system.

A definite benefit is obtained when all dietary antigens derived from foods are removed by fasting. When patients with rheumatoid arthritis are allowed only water on a seven- to ten-day fast, joint pains are substantially reduced and stiffness decreases. Fasting also reduces inflammation by altering excessive activities attributed to the white blood cells and other components of the immune system.

Over time, the markers of inflammation in the blood invariably fall as the fast progresses. For example, the erythrocyte sedimentation rate (ESR) falls to about 5, well within the normal range.

When fasting, the intestinal tract has the opportunity to become quiet, which in turn gives the immune system a much needed rest. Fasting not only stops the input of all potential protein antigens and food-derived toxins, but also allows the digestive tract to rest and heal, restoring its structural integrity. After the fast, the system will not be as sensitive to potential food allergens because of decreased amounts of potential immune-stimulating peptides crossing the mucosal defenses.

Another positive aspect of the fast is its ability to increase microcirculation to the joints. The negative nutrition associated with fasting mobilizes the fat stores of the entire body, including the pathologic fat stores lining vessels in the macro- and micro-circulation, thus supplying the joints with a more adequate oxygen supply. This in turn enables the elimination of retained waste in the joint capsule and allows the inflammation in the joints to subside. In this manner the body is able to catch up on its internal housecleaning, and retained antibody–antigen complexes are eliminated from the joints and connective tissue. Thus the remarkable self-repairing process of the fast begins by removing the triggers to immune hypersensitivity.

Fasting has been shown not only to reduce inflammation, swelling, and pain in arthritis sufferers, but also to enhance the ability of the immune system to fight infection.[23] The studies done on fasting for autoimmune diseases have consistently shown multiple benefits to the arthritic, especially when combined with a dairy-free, vegetarian diet.[24,25] Some of these studies were carefully done in a crossover manner in which the examiners did not know which patients were in the fasted group.

Another important reason fasting is able to ameliorate the clinical manifestations of rheumatoid arthritis is that it alters the fatty acid composition of cellular membranes, taking away important triggers to the autoimmune inflammatory process. This positive effect of fasting has been studied and explained in detail in the scientific literature on fasting.[26] It is remarkable to watch the pain, stiffness, and swelling melt away as the fast progresses. The predictability of this response is dramatic. It is exceedingly rare that we do not see dramatic improvement that most often results in complete freedom from pain by the time the fast is completed.

Clearly, when a properly conducted fast is combined with an optimal dietary approach for each individual, the patient has the greatest chance of achieving a total clinical remission.

The results of a study comparing two groups of patients who

were tracked for one year were published in the October 12, 1991, issue of *The Lancet*, a respected medical journal. The control group was treated with the conventional medical approach, utilizing drugs. The other group received no medication and was placed on a seven- to ten-day partial fast, followed by a low-fat, dairy-free, plant-based diet. The results, carefully monitored by blood tests and physician examiners, documented the vast superiority of the dietary approach. All clinical examinations were done by a physician who did not know the group to which the patient had been allocated.

Food was reintroduced after the fast very gradually, which is important in achieving consistent results in such patients. A "new" food item was introduced every second day. If a patient noticed an increase in pain, stiffness, or joint swelling within 48 hours, the item was omitted from the diet for at least seven days. If symptoms were exacerbated on reintroduction of this food, it was excluded from the diet for the rest of the study period.

The patients in the control group treated with drugs ate ordinary food. In the intervention group, in the first three to five months after the fast the patients were asked not to eat food that contained gluten, meat, fish, eggs, dairy products, refined sugar, citrus fruits, salt, strong spices, preservatives, alcohol, tea, and coffee.

After four weeks the intervention group showed a significant improvement in the number of tender joints, pain score, morning stiffness, and grip strength. The blood markers of inflammation, including the erythrocyte sedimentation rate (ESR) and C-reactive protein also showed significant improvement.

The benefits to the fasting–diet group were still present after one year. The evaluation of the whole course showed significant advantages for the fasting–diet group in all measured indicators.[27]

These studies corroborate the clinical evidence of doctors utilizing this approach to autoimmune disease, and the experience of thousands of patients who have recovered their health through natural diet and fasting. In fact, there are so many carefully done studies in the scientific literature on this subject[28] that the conventionally held viewpoints should be considered irresponsible, bordering on medical malpractice, since this nutritional approach is safe, potentially curative, and may save the patient from a lifetime of toxic drugs. Yet there is a mere handful of physicians at this time who practice this approach.

In the *Medical Tribune,*[29] a publication read by a great number of American physicians, I recently noted a report documenting the beneficial effect of a vegetable diet on autoimmune diseases including lupus, arthritis, and nephrotic syndrome. A few months later in the same medical periodical I read an article in which a rheumatologist stated that diet plays no role in the treatment of rheumatoid arthritis. He stated, "It cannot be proven that diet influences this disease."[30] I was reminded of all the proclamations over the last thirty years stating that it cannot be proven that smoking causes lung cancer.

A week after reading the rheumatologist's statement I wrote the following letter to the editor, which appeared in the *Medical Tribune* of December 10, 1992.

Don't Ignore the Diet in Arthritis

The recent article on state-of-the-art treatment for arthritis restated the generally held opinion that diet plays no role in the treatment of rheumatoid arthritis.

This is in spite of studies which document the effectiveness of specific diets, studies even reported in the *Medical Tribune.*[31] One recent study placed patients with severe arthritis on a fast for 7–10 days, and then followed up with a low-fat, gluten and dairy-free, plant-based diet. They then compared the results with the control group that was treated with traditional medical protocols, including powerful drugs. The diet approach was far superior in getting results.[32]

I see the same impressive results when my patients try these dietary approaches. I'll give one case history out of many.

A 62-year-old woman with severe rheumatoid arthritis and other problems was on nine different medications—Altace,

Azulfidine, Beclovent, digoxin, Ecotrin, Nasalchrome, Organidine, prednisone, and Seldane. She hadn't been able to close her hand to make a fist in 10 years and had pain in multiple joints.

Despite visiting numerous physicians and having received almost all of the treatments mentioned in the article on arthritis, she was still getting worse. We decided to begin a fast, followed by a plant-based vegetarian diet. After the medically supervised fast the arthritis was gone.

Her ESR had dropped from 42 (on prednisone) to 13 (off prednisone) and she is still on the diet now, five months later. She has continued to remain free of symptoms. She no longer requires any of the nine medications she had needed before coming to my office six months ago. She has regained the physical strength and movement that was lost over 10 years ago.

In addition, she has lost 35 pounds, her high blood pressure and other medical problems have resolved.

In these days of methotrexate, gold salts, steroids, and the other big guns in our medical arsenal of treatments, it might seem preposterous that something as simple as diet might benefit arthritis. However, in light of the results that are now documented with plant-based diets, I consider statements rebutting the role diet plays in the treatment of arthritis to be ill-informed and perhaps irresponsible.

Joel Fuhrman, M.D.
Belle Mead, N.J.

After this letter appeared, I received numerous enthusiastic calls from other physicians around the country, requesting further information, corroborating my findings, and referring me their patients.

Psoriasis

Psoriasis and psoriatic arthritis also respond favorably to the combination of fasting and dietary intervention. In one medical study, eight out of ten patients noted improvement in their psoriasis after a short fast (seven to ten days).[33] My experience has shown that most patients' psoriatic lesions improve if they fast long enough. Substantial results often require a long fast (14 to 30 days), maintenance of a thin body, and a careful diet after the fast is completed.

I frequently note that when people with psoriasis and eczema fast, the results of their liver-function tests routinely elevate early and then normalize as the fast is taken to completion. Without the normalization of the liver from the detoxifying effect of a more prolonged fast (three to five weeks), reappearance of skin lesions may occur upon reintroduction of food. Invariably when the psoriasis sufferer overeats and puts on too much fat after fasting, the problem once again emerges.

Systemic Lupus Erythematosus

Systemic lupus erythematosus (SLE), or simply lupus, as it is often called, is yet another autoimmune disease with serious consequences. A variety of body systems may be involved, including joints, the skin, and the kidneys. Excessive female sex hormones, particularly estrogen, influence the immune system, making females more susceptible to lupus. There is an increased chance of developing lupus during pregnancy or with the use of birth control pills because these are situations in which estrogen levels increase dramatically.

While conventional therapy with steroids and cytotoxic agents can help to control symptoms, it does not treat their underlying cause. Unfortunately, the scientific literature is biased toward chemotherapeutic agents, which produce severe side effects, rather than "unconventional" treatments such as dietary modification.[34] I can usually spot the lupus sufferers as they walk into

159

my office. After years of taking dangerous steroids such as prednisone, their bodies are swollen like balloons.

Recent evidence suggests that certain foods are common offenders in aggravating the symptoms of lupus. Understandably, the reactivity of autoantibodies in lupus sufferers strongly cross-reacts with commonly ingested animal proteins. Blood serum from those with SLE can also react with proteins from plants. These proteins can be found in soy beans, corn, spinach, and carrots.[35] Though the animal-food-based proteins are the prime offenders, this indicates that occasionally plant foods should be tested for immune reactivity as well.

Alfalfa sprouts are also to be avoided in cases of lupus because ingestion of alfalfa seed sprouts or L-canavanine, a prominent constituent of alfalfa, causes SLE-like diseases in primates.[36,37] L-canavanine is also present in other legumes, or beans, so these, too, often need to be avoided.

Lupus flare-ups have also been reported after ingestion of large amounts of foods containing psoralens (celery, celery salt, parsnips, figs).[38] Psoralens are chemicals that increase photosensitivity in those who are sun-sensitive. Hydrazines, the chemicals believed responsible for many cases of drug-induced lupus, are also present in mushrooms, some food dyes, tobacco smoke, and most cooked foods, especially cooked meats and other fatty foods.

Hair dyes contain high levels of hydrazines and other related chemicals that are absorbed through the scalp. People exposed to hair dyes also have a significantly increased risk of lupus.[39,40]

Dr. Paul Agris, a physician researcher on lupus and food sensitivities, has noted numerous physicians who have described cases in which patients with SLE have had dietary modifications influence the way they feel and the severity of their lupus symptoms.[41] The foods typically involved animal-based foods, not plant products.

The evidence of the powerful role diet plays in SLE and other autoimmune and collagen vascular disease stems from multiple animal studies. These studies note how mice and other animals with lupus fed a low-fat diet had significantly lower ANA positivity (a marker of disease activity in the blood) and improved survival, when compared to animals with lupus on a higher fat diet.[42,43]

Not only have certain fats been implicated by animal studies, but also some proteins, especially cow's milk proteins, have been strongly implicated in lupus and other autoimmune illnesses. Interestingly, mice with lupus live many times longer when their diet is free of cow's milk.[44]

Beef and milk are probably the most offensive of all foods to the lupus sufferer, and are repeatedly implicated in investigations.[45] Animal products typically combine a high-protein content with a high-fat content, a combination inadvisable to those suffering with autoimmune illness. Vegetable oils should also be eliminated from the lupus diet. This is because any fat—whether derived from animal or plant—increases body fat and the level of circulating estrogen, and this too contributes to the immune malfunction in lupus.

As soon as a person is diagnosed with lupus, he or she should immediately begin a medically supervised fast to initiate a remission. Breaking the fast carefully under proper guidance is extremely important. Upon completion of the fast the following foods should be avoided for a prolonged period of time:

1. All animal foods, including dairy and eggs
2. All legumes, except for peas and lima beans
3. Celery, corn, alfalfa sprouts, mushrooms, spinach, and figs.

Exposure to all chemicals should be carefully avoided as well. Specifically, avoid cigarette smoke, hair dyes, and pesticides. All plant food should be organically grown or pesticide-free.

The fundamental problem in lupus seems to be that once autoantibody production is triggered, it fails to shut down. This is the case even after the removal of potentially inciting factors.

Many lupus sufferers make autoantibodies against their own suppressor T cells. This causes innumerable problems because suppressor T cells are the cells that can modulate or turn off the immune response. A vicious cycle is thereby created. Unrestrained by suppressor T cells, antibodies flourish and destroy more tissues, more suppressor T cells, and so on. This is why a fast is needed, and is especially important early in the disease because fasting can turn off this self-destructive autoimmune process. The fast allows the body to finally turn down the triggered, revved-up immune system that is out of control. Then, when an appropriate diet is followed after the fast, the patient can stay well.

It is very difficult to inhibit this vicious cycle by dietary change alone, though it does occur in some people. A good example is the case reported in *The Lancet* of a 16-year-old girl with a continually worsening condition in spite of aggressive steroid therapy. Against her physician's advice, she tapered herself off the steroids and embarked on a healthy, well-planned vegetarian diet. In a short time, her antibody titers (indicators of disease activity) normalized, urinary protein excretion decreased, and serum albumin rose.[46]

When a physician pays close attention to the *causes* of lupus and concentrates on detoxification through fasting and diet, the results are predictable. However, when the disease has advanced and the patient has been taking toxic medication for years, the results are more unpredictable and less favorable. Even so, a natural approach should still be tried in advanced cases because improvement and even remissions are still possible.

Sarah, a 37-year-old woman, was diagnosed with lupus in 1987. Since her diagnosis she had been treated with numerous potent medications to suppress inflammation. She did not improve, however. By 1992 she suffered from neurological complications (headaches, dizziness, loss of balance, and nausea). She also complained of joint and chest pain. Frustrated by her deteriorating condition, and upon the recommendation of a friend who was familiar with my approach to treating autoimmune disease, she made an appointment to see me.

After undergoing a 20-day fast in the fall of 1992, Sarah was placed on a low-fat, low-protein diet, specifically devoid of dairy products. Although initially weak from her underlying disease and the fast, she rapidly regained her strength. She was now off all medications and all her lupus symptoms had resolved. Moreover, her lupus antibody level and ANA titer (a measure of disease activity), both previously high, tested normal.

Though this approach might seem highly unusual to some, it is not only safer than the current treatments, but also, when started early in the disease process, can offer complete remission from the disease. The patient can live a completely normal life free of both the effects of the disease and the effects of the toxic drug treatments.

Dorothy, a 43-year-old woman with lupus for more than ten years, was on five different medications when she first came to my office. Her prednisone (a steroid medication) dose had recently been raised to 25 mg. by her rheumatologist because she had had continual flairs with stabbing chest pain, joint pains, and skin rashes. She also had significant anemia and a rapid heartbeat. During the first month, we gradually discontinued her medications so she could begin a fast.

After a person has been on steroid medication for such a long time, extreme caution must be followed during the fast because their adrenal function will still be suppressed from the chronic use of steroid medications. For this reason and because of her rapid heart rate, Dorothy was fasted for only one week. I was unsure whether this short a fast would offer her significant results, given the severity of her condition.

A few weeks later, Dorothy informed me that her joint pain was gone. Two months later she was back to full-time work, for the first time in many years. She needed no medication. She felt great and was exercising and lifting weights and looked like a completely new person. We were both thrilled with her results.

The underlying cause of disease must be treated whenever possible. While the specific etiology of lupus even now is still not well defined, there is sufficient evidence to attempt this most conservative, safe, and ultimately effective approach before using the "big guns," such as steroids and chemotherapeutic drugs, which have numerous hazardous side effects. If a patient is treated early enough with this nondrug approach, drug-based treatment of lupus can usually be eliminated.

Inflammatory Bowel Disease: Ulcerative Colitis and Crohn's Disease

Ulcerative colitis and Crohn's disease are inflammatory diseases involving the lining of the intestines. They are considered idiopathic, meaning that the cause of the disease is unknown. Colitis involves the large intestine, or colon. It is accompanied by pain and loose stools that can contain blood and mucus. Crohn's disease affects mostly young adults. Separate areas of the bowel can be ulcerated or inflamed though other segments between the ulcerations can be unaffected.

The abnormal interaction between the immune system and the digestive tract causes these diseases to evolve. Rarely, colitis may be caused by infection, and anyone with inflammatory bowel disease should initially undergo appropriate stool analysis to rule out infectious causes such as parasites or bacterial pathogens.

Patients with these physically and emotionally devastating diseases may have as many as 20 bloody bowel movements daily. Sometimes, even the strongest medications cannot help.

As with other autoimmune disease, inflammatory bowel disease is common in the developed countries. This is clearly related to the animal food and cow's-milk-rich diet we feed ourselves and especially our children. How we are fed at a young age is crucially important and can have a profound effect on our future health.

In recent decades the incidence of irritable bowel disease has rapidly increased in our children.[47] Rather than raising infants as nature designed on an early diet exclusively of breast milk with the later addition of natural plant foods, many parents raise their children primarily on substances that breed illness: formula, then sugary foods, bottled fruit juices, processed foods, cow's milk, and other high-fat animal products.

Prolonged breast-feeding and the delayed introduction of other foods in other countries may point to the cause of our own high incidence of autoimmune illnesses and especially inflammatory bowel disease. It is well established that the digestive tract in the bottle-fed infant is exposed to insults from potentially pathogenic microorganisms and offensive food antigens. The rich levels of secretory IgA (an immunoglobulin) in mother's milk protect against these digestive problems.[48] Therefore, the continuation of breast-feeding when solid food is first introduced is especially important in the second half of the child's first year.

The damage from our aberrant infant feeding practices in this country cannot be overemphasized. It has been repeatedly noted in the medical literature that the exposure to cow's milk (a food obviously designed for infant cows, not humans) increases the risk not only of adverse reactions to this milk, but also of developing allergies to other foods.[49]

Potentially damaging cow's milk proteins are also present in many cow's-milk-based infant formulas. In the genetically sensitive individual, the lack of breast-feeding or abbreviated breast-feeding, combined with the early introduction of cow's milk, could significantly contribute to the later development of inflammatory bowel disease.

Cow's milk protein has been implicated as a causative factor in ulcerative colitis for more than three decades.[50,51] In some clinical trials, remission and relapse were correlated with milk intake.[52] Scientific investigations have illustrated that cow's milk proteins are so inflammatory in ulcerative colitis patients that the way in which lymphocytes react to cow's milk may serve as a marker of active disease.[53]

Obviously, it is important for all inflammatory bowel disease sufferers to avoid any and all dairy products. The harmful and disease-producing effects of cow's-milk-based food fed to our infants span the broad spectrum of autoimmune diseases, frequent infection, and decreased immunity to disease in general. Milk is a contributing factor to all the other diseases mentioned in this chapter, as well as to ulcerative colitis.

Evidence now suggests that the increased intake of dietary sugars, acetaminophen, and other non-narcotic analgesics may also exacerbate Crohn's disease.[54] Therefore, the intake of refined sugars, or too many sweet fruits, may also need to be carefully monitored in those with Crohn's disease or other autoimmune diseases.

If we exceed the capacity of our digestive apparatus to absorb sugar, the unabsorbed sugars can be fermented by bacterial action lower down in the gut, forming acetic acid, lactic acid, alcohol, and other irritating products. Both sucrose and gluten have been implicated in inflammatory bowel disease for decades.[55,56] One reason for this may be the way these elements affect bacterial activity in the gut. Therefore, it is often necessary for patients to religiously avoid breads and cereals in order to completely remove from their diet gluten that is contained in grains such as wheat, barley, oats, and rye.

Clearly no specific diet is appropriate for all patients. The diet must be always modified to the severity of the illness and the uniqueness of each individual.

When the disease is relatively mild or takes a mild form—such as proctitis—often all that is needed is a change in diet that eliminates sugar, fats, oils, and dairy products. When the disease is more extensive and aggressive, however, more broad dietary intervention is needed.

Elimination diets have repeatedly been shown to be beneficial to those with any type of autoimmune illness. An elimination diet begins with either a fast or with eating only a few foods. Gradually, other foods are added, usually only one new food daily, and then that food is eliminated if it triggers a reaction or causes additional symptoms. One study of inflammatory bowel disease patients who followed elimination diet regimens reported a remission rate of 62 percent after one year and a cumulative remission rate of 45 percent after five years.[57]

Exclusion diets have also been studied and shown to be highly effective in those with Crohn's disease.[58] An exclusion diet consists of only a liquid that has in it vitamins, minerals, glucose, and

166

water, but no food. It is like a partial fast. In one study, after 14 days on the supplemented fast, 78 of the 93 patients (84 percent) achieved remission. Those who achieved remission with this partial fast were then split into two groups. One group received further treatment with prednisone and the other group was slowly reintroduced to foods. Only a single new food was introduced per day. Any food that provoked symptoms of diarrhea or pain was thereafter excluded. The researchers found intolerance to many foods in various patients. These foods included corn, wheat, milk, yeast, egg, potato, rye, apples, mushrooms, and oats. Coffee, tea, and chocolate were also revealed as exciting factors.

Relapses occurred in 66 percent of the steroid-treated group, while only 30 percent of those treated with the elimination diet showed any signs of recurrence. This study corroborated my personal experience that each patient's special needs and individual tolerances need to be taken into consideration at all times.

Frequently, when the disease is active and there is bleeding, individuals cannot tolerate any uncooked food. They are best fed with stewed or steamed vegetables exclusively. Persons who are actively bleeding should consume a diet of soft (steamed or stewed) vegetables until they can embark upon a fast. The diet should be composed of vegetables such as stewed zucchini, sweet potato, squash, and new potatoes (no skin). All food should be chewed exceptionally well. No fruit juices, citrus fruits, or tomatoes should be eaten; even other fruits may need to be avoided. Avoid cereals and all grains except for well-cooked rice. Raw vegetable juice (cabbage or lettuce juice with a little carrot juice added) is usually nonirritating. Taking large amounts of essential fatty acids, such as flax oil, borage oil, evening primrose oil, or fish oils, is sometimes helpful as a natural anti-inflammatory to help patients avoid or lessen the need for medication.

Fasting should not be avoided in those with Crohn's disease, even if they respond to the above dietary changes without fasting. Fasting is an important element if a sustained remission is to be expected. The fast allows the entire system to restore its cellular and immunogenic integrity. The inflamed bowel can rest and heal because the main irritant to the system—food—is withdrawn.

With any autoimmune illness, fasting should be employed at the earliest possible point. In many instances, however, fasting must be delayed until the patient is slowly tapered off medications. During this period prior to the fast, the inflammatory bowel disease sufferer should be eating primarily stewed, baked, and steamed vegetables.

Once an adequate remission has been obtained from the use of the modified diet in conjunction with an extended fast, foods should be introduced very gradually, beginning with the stewed and baked vegetables that we used before the fast. In time, the diet can gradually be broadened to include more raw and high-fiber fruit, vegetables, and grains. Nuts, seeds, and legumes may be consumed sparingly. Later on, after a remission has been induced, high-fiber diets have actually been shown to be of definite benefit.[59,60]

A physician experienced in caring for these patients through nutritional means can obtain excellent results in minimizing or avoiding the use of toxic drugs, such as prednisone, and preventing radical bowel surgery, which is so often performed in these cases.

One of my patients has a strong family history of ulcerative colitis. She and all of her siblings have the disease. She fasted for three weeks to place the disease in remission. Now she undergoes an extended fast every few years to ensure that she maintains her remission. Periodically, we order blood tests to check for markers of inflammation even though she is well and has no symptoms. In this manner, we can detect early signs that a flare-up may occur and then, if indicated, she can begin another fast before an actual flare-up of the disease develops.

Superior Nutrition Is Essential After the Fast

One of the reasons why certain diets have not been shown to be universally successful with autoimmune diseases is that just eliminating a few foods from the pitiful American diet is not sufficient. Also, there is no particular diet that is just right for everyone. Each patient may need certain modifications to avoid consuming foods that excite an excessive immune response and those they do not digest well.

Sometimes patients with severely leaky guts may have to avoid certain foods that may be perfectly fine for another patient with the same illness. For example, a very small percentage of arthritis patients note that their condition is worsened by the consumption of foods in the nightshade family, such as tomatoes, peppers, eggplant, and white potatoes. Citrus fruits or wheat products are also common offenders. The foods that need to be avoided can often be identified by blood or urine testing.

Ferric nitrate urine testing can be useful to help identify foods that are not digested properly. During this test, the person eats only one food; then the first urine passed after that meal is tested to see how much sediment it contains. One can learn how efficient digestion of that particular food was, and whether or not the body was flooded by immune complex formation after eating it. In this manner we can customize the diet to ensure it is the best possible one for each.

A review of the scientific literature regarding autoimmune disease and food allergy shows that patients consistently improve when care is taken to customize a diet through elimination of those foods that may be sensitizing for that individual. The improvement is often striking when the proper diet is designed individually for each patient.[61] Very often researchers first employ the fast in their treatment because fasting is well known to bring about a quick remission of symptoms.[62] Once the symptoms are improved or resolved as a result of the fast, it is easier for the physician and the patient to determine which foods can exacerbate the pain. By carefully reintroducing foods slowly, one at a time, and by eliminating any food that causes an increase in symptoms, each individual can recognize optimal nutrition.

The human body contains powerful self-remedying forces. If we can unleash this healing potential by removing the causes of illness and remove all impediments to healing, the results can be truly remarkable.

The greatest enemy to healing is the well-meaning physician who initially starts the patient with autoimmune disease on powerful drugs. Treatments build complications and prolong the illness so that the sufferer now has multiple reasons for systemic toxicity. One also should be in touch with his or her body to know if overeating, insufficient rest, or dietary indiscretions will cause symptoms. Through healthful living and avoiding suppression of early symptoms with drugs, we can avoid the development of chronic disease or the return to the former disease condition once a recovery has been achieved.

The sooner a person is placed on drugs, including the stronger and more toxic medications, the more difficult and prolonged is the healing process when he or she finally decides to get off the drugging merry-go-round.

Massage, hot baths, herbs, mineral salts, acupuncture, serums, and electric therapies have all been found to be ineffective, though some have afforded temporary relief, because no true healing can take place unless the causes of ill health are removed. The primary cause of illness can be summed up in one word: toxicosis. The self-pollution that destroys our bodies from the inside out, from wrong living and wrong eating, is a dangerous life-style to continue.

Unfortunately, many patients have been drugged and treated for so long that by the time they are ready or aware that there is a way to get well from their condition, they already have skeletal deformity, fused joints, and some degree of irreparable damage.

That doesn't mean we can't improve their condition, but by failing to use this nutritional approach earlier, they have denied themselves the ability to achieve a complete remission of their illness.

Many of the people who are taking multiple medications when they first seek my services cannot be placed on a fast initially. First, we must decrease their dependency on medication. Tapering medications such as prednisone may take many weeks while they are improving from the dietary change. We utilize the fast at a later stage when they can more comfortably stop their medications.

Sometimes I recommend natural anti-inflammatory substances, which do not have the same toxicity as drugs, to help us taper off the medication. These natural anti-inflammatories include fish oils, borage oil, and flax oil, taken either alone or in combination, to help lessen the need for more toxic drugs. These can be especially useful in reducing the need for prednisone in arthritis and colitis patients, and have been shown in multiple studies to do so.[63] Other nutrients, such as fructo-oligosaccharides, and beneficial bacteria are occasionally indicated to help enhance the healing of mucosal epithelial tissue.[64]

One of my patients with severe rheumatoid arthritis appeared to be doing very well. She exhibited less and less joint pain as she followed the diet I had prepared for her. We slowly tapered her prednisone and other drugs over a three-month period. About one week after she was finally off all drugs, she phoned to tell me she had suffered a severe flare-up of her condition, and was immobile in almost every joint in her body. She was ready to give up and go back on prednisone at this time. Fortunately, I convinced her that this was the time to begin her fast. Her symptoms resolved quickly while fasting and now, years later, she has never had a reoccurrence of her rheumatoid arthritis symptoms.

If the fast is followed by a low-protein, natural food, vegetarian diet and the individual avoids irritating foods that have been found to cause the immune system to over-react, he or she can be forever cured of the autoimmune illness. Fasting is the starting point. It should be thought of as the initial preparation of housecleaning before embarking on a new way of eating and living that will support health and not cause the body to break down again.

Many people will feel this approach is too sacrificial, that it requires too much discipline, or takes too long. Some are looking for instantaneous health, so they continue to search for "cures" that don't exist. However, the people I see generally state they are "sick of being sick" and are glad to finally get to the bottom of their conditions and attempt to remove the cause. They don't find the diet restrictive, as there is sufficient variety among their choices. Rather, they enjoy the foods and their new-found health. They usually show determination and a positive enthusiasm, and accordingly earn the desired results.

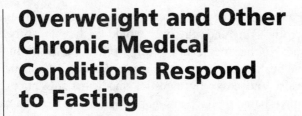

8 Overweight and Other Chronic Medical Conditions Respond to Fasting

> This is the first time I have felt well since my honeymoon.
> I finally have control and insight as to my own body. I feel
> young and beautiful again. Thank you, Dr. Fuhrman.
>
> —P. Reile

Fasting Is Effective for a Large Variety of Ailments

I was fortunate enough to be exposed to the benefits of fasting
when I was very young. I have been able to observe its usefulness
over the years for thousands of people. Today, there are a mere
handful of physicians practicing this approach in the country. But
many patients with grave conditions seek this type of help after
all other approaches have failed. First, though, they embarked on
another journey, spending years searching for and seeing all the
top specialists in the field, and spending huge sums of money.
They tried various drugging treatments, yet still became worse.
They hadn't yet come to the understanding that drugs do not
remove the cause of disease, and they were given more and more
toxic substances to ingest by well-meaning physicians. While these
drugs were consumed in hope of lessening their symptoms, the
causes of disease continued to press on with their nefarious influence, allowing the disease to progress and worsen. Then, they
often spent many more thousands of dollars on alternative practitioners and were given more "cures" to no avail. Finally, after
years of searching, these determined but still suffering individuals
were told there is a method of care based on human physiology,
and they decided to try it as a last resort.

Unlike other methods of disease treatment, fasting is not based on giving cures, because to expect a cure or remedy to undo years of wrong living and self-abuse would be the same as believing in magic. Neither magic, nor getting something for nothing, works in the health and disease care arena. We cannot suspend the laws of cause and effect by ingesting medicinal substances. Instead, fasting is based on unchanging biological laws that insist the cause of disease be removed.

After hearing about a natural food diet and therapeutic fasting, individuals may enthusiastically give it a try and get well. It is also possible that they may become excited about the sensibleness of this approach and the prospect of finally recovering their health, but then go home to their friends and family and become discouraged after being told that they would be crazy to attempt such an "outrageous" treatment. They might even call a few doctors they know only to be told that fasting is risky, dangerous, and stupid.

It continually amazes me how "expert" opinions can be given on something with which someone has had no experience, knows nothing about, and has never researched. I once had occasion to speak to one such well-meaning physician who was furiously opposed to fasting. I told him I had read, and was thoroughly familiar with, more than five hundred medical journal articles on therapeutic fasting. I inquired as to which ones he was familiar with to help him reach his opinion. His answer was that he had not read any of them. He actually had zero knowledge about the subject and began to ask me questions. He was consumed with the same vague fears and questions the typical layman would have. Though still having doubts, after our conversation he admitted he had given his opinion too hastily, and had much more to learn.

The physicians who regularly utilize therapeutic fasting in their practice see so many remarkable recoveries that getting well is the expected, the normal outcome. This is because nature heals when given the opportunity.

Still, despite these studies on fasting and plant-based diets, the world largely ignores this treatment because it is contrary to the present system of medical practice. Doctors would have to remodel their entire approach to health and disease, and many physicians would have to admit that most of what they do is not needed or useful. This is not going to happen soon. We must expect powerful opposition to the method of care presented here.

Too often, scientific experiments prove nothing. Frequently, the source of the money dictates the answer. Yet these experiments are all we have to go by and are crucially important when we are testing potentially dangerous drugs that may have various hazardous effects. Fasting and adopting an optimal diet designed to aid one's condition, on the other hand, are health supporting. They will make a healthy person even healthier.

Most physicians who have knowledge and expertise in therapeutic fasting advise it for those wishing to maintain their body in optimal health and to extend life. It is not merely for the sick. Many of these physicians, including myself, have personally undertaken long fasts, and may do so periodically. For example, Dr. Alec Burton, an osteopathic physician who has fasted more than thirty thousand patients, undergoes a two-week fast every few years for the long-term health benefits that accrue from the rejuvenating effects of the fast. I too, plan to undergo another fast in the near future even though I am in excellent health.

The point I am making is that fasting improves one's health, rather than insults it with dangerous drugs or unnecessary and potentially deadly surgery. If fasting does not lead to complete recovery from a certain condition, it will not hurt you, either, and will actually improve your health.

Patients who choose this method of care generally become the most enthusiastic supporters of fasting once they have undergone the experience. They are excited to have avoided surgery or a lifetime of drug use. Many different conditions are aided by fasting, a few of which I shall discuss in this chapter.

Using Fasting to Conquer Uterine Fibroids

When I fasted my first patient with uterine fibroids, and watched the tumor shrink by 78 percent after two weeks of the fast, even

I was surprised by how effective fasting was for this condition. In Randi's case, we knew that prior to the fast the tumor had been getting larger with more severe bleeding for years. Many physicians encouraged her to have it surgically removed. Randi chose to fast instead.

Pelvic ultrasounds done by a radiologist both before and after Randi's fast documented the cubic size of the tumor and the exact percent of shrinkage that occurred. Her fibroid tumor measured 473.6 cubic centimeters before the 14-day fast and 105.8 cubic centimeters after. Of additional note was that this patient also had rosacea, a chronic distressing skin condition with extreme redness around the nose and cheeks. The rosacea disappeared with fasting and did not return.

More than half a million women have hysterectomies each year. Many of them experience depression, painful intercourse, and urinary problems after surgery. Fasting not only allows the fibroid to shrink, but also often sets into motion a process in which the fibroid continues to shrink after the fast. The pain and pressure from fibroids and the excessive bleeding predictably respond to this method of care. Avoiding unnecessary surgery is precisely why many patients choose to undergo a therapeutic fast.

Using Fasting to Conquer Benign Tumors

Fasting is a safe and effective approach for not only fibroid tumors, but also most noncancerous tumors. Nasal polyps, lipomas, benign ovarian tumors, and benign tumors of the breast often respond favorably to therapeutic fasting, especially when the person is not very overweight.

When an individual has lots of fat on his or her body, the likelihood of reducing a tumor through fasting is uncertain because the body will likely use the fat stores as the primary energy source rather than the tumor. The best way to utilize fasting to shrink a benign tumor in severely overweight persons is for them to adopt an excellent diet and exercise program for some months prior to fasting. After they are in better shape, they can undertake the fast and expect more predictable results.

Fasting can also be utilized to aid in the diagnosis of a suspicious mass such as an ovarian tumor. Since noncancerous or benign ovarian tumors typically respond rapidly to a fast, one may undertake a fast and then recheck with ultrasound to see if the tumor has shrunk. If, after a ten- to fourteen-day fast, the tumor stays the same size, then it is more likely that the mass may represent cancer and should be surgically removed.

Cancerous tumors should not be expected to respond to a fast. If a cancerous tumor does shrink or disappear because of fasting, it is most likely it was not cancer to begin with, and the diagnosis should be carefully reconsidered. Generally, fasting should not be recommended for patients with cancer. An individual with advanced cancer may be advised to fast, not to improve his or her condition, but to lessen pain and hasten death. When a person is suffering from advanced disease and will soon die, he or she may die more comfortably while fasting.

Cancers are generally unregulated growths. Their behavior is uncontrolled, and the cells multiply rapidly, disseminate (metastasize), and invade surrounding structures. Factors such as hormones, adequacy of blood supply, and various unknown influences can affect their growth. Noncancerous tissue, on the other hand, is more responsive to bodily control because benign tumors behave more predictably, are generally more slow to grow, and follow normal rules. The nutritional and hormonal changes that occur in the fasting state, especially as body fat stores are largely depleted, cause the body to recognize noncancerous tumors and target and tap them as a source of extra (unessential) tissue for nourishment. The body has less influence over the behavior of cancerous tumors, which often seem to have their own, independent agenda.

Sometimes even relatively minor chronic conditions can be troublesome to a patient—conditions such as recurrent or chronic sinusitis and allergies. Even when these conditions become advanced and patients are advised to undergo sinus surgery, I routinely watch them rid themselves of the problem by adopting the fasting/optimal diet approach.

One patient who came to me had been advised to have sinus surgery the following week for chronic congestion and obliteration of his left sinus cavity, as demonstrated on a CT scan. He had been complaining of allergic rhinitis, facial pain, and troubling congestion for years. He came to me for a second opinion in the hope of avoiding surgery. I suggested we delay surgery for a few weeks and try a more conservative natural approach first, to see if it would help.

Thinking he had nothing to lose, he agreed, but felt he would still require surgery within a few months. The plan was for him to undergo a fast in two or three months after following a nontoxic, high-antioxidant diet to maximize his immune response. At the follow-up visit one month later, before he fasted, he noted his symptoms had significantly lessened. In fact, by the time I saw him at the next follow-up one month later, his symptoms had completely resolved, his CT scan had normalized, and he did not need to fast. Obviously, his condition was not resistant enough to require a fast. He decided to continue the healthy diet and was pleased with the results. Fasting can be very helpful for cases of resistant sinus congestion, and can even shrink nasal polyps.

Asthma also predictably responds to fasting, and it does so in resistant cases in which even medication cannot adequately control symptoms. Asthma has an inflammatory and possibly an autoimmune component and could even be compared to the diseases mentioned in Chapter 7.

Many diseases of an "allergic" nature represent an oversensitivity of the immune system. It is always prudent to remove known allergens in the sensitive individual. However, when does anyone consider why this individual is so hypersensitive or allergic? Improving one's health can enable allergies to resolve. It's exciting to see someone eating and enjoying a food that they hadn't been able to eat in years because of food allergies. This happens routinely on the fast; allergies simply go away as the person's health improves.

The hyper-reactivity of the asthmatic's airways may be caused by sensitivity to allergens, and may also be brought on by infections, irritants, exercise, or even emotions. Yet in every case there is an underlying abnormality—an irritability of the airway that leads to inflammation, spasm, and narrowing of the air passages. This excessive irritability decreases and even resolves when the body is allowed to detoxify through fasting.

It is also well established that some medications used to treat asthma, while giving short-term relief, actually worsen the condition in the long run and increase the risk of asthma-related death.[1,2] The discontinuance of these medications can improve asthma control. Only through aggressive nutritional management can the individual's overall health improve enough so that less asthma medication is utilized.

The more severe the asthma and the greater the dependency on medication, the longer it takes to achieve a recovery when we apply natural methods. Establishing a complete recovery for the severely asthmatic patient can be relatively difficult compared to many other diseases, but perseverance pays off. I have found that a long fast, or sometimes two fasts with impeccable dietary habits in between, is usually essential for the resolution when the patient has been dependent on multiple medications for many years.

The beneficial effects of fasting in asthmatics have been well documented in the Russian medical literature.[3,4] One recent study concluded that fasting is the only nonmedical way to improve asthma control. After observing the results obtained from many years of collecting case histories and reviewing other studies, Russian physicians concluded that fasting should be considered the treatment of choice in patients with complicated, serious bronchial asthma.[5] They reported that fasting not only decreased the allergic inflammatory process, but also increased resistance and immunity to bacterial infections. Their clinical trials illustrated that more than 75 percent of patients had greatly improved conditions or never had symptoms of asthma again after fasting.

Fasting and natural diet should be the treatment of choice for all asthmatics. A rare exception to this would be asthma symptoms caused by a toxic exposure, such as occupational asthma, where all that is needed for recovery is identifying and removing the offending substance. We should not wait until any disease becomes so severe that it is difficult to remedy when a safe and more effective method of restoring normal function, like fasting, can be utilized.

One must recognize that, as with all diseases, many years of drugging takes its toll: the longer the patient waits to utilize this effective natural approach, the more difficult it will be and the longer it will take to bring about a recovery.

Of course there are limitations to what one fast can do. Occasionally, when the fast is trying to address many years of self-abuse, the patient either is not willing to fast long enough to achieve a complete recovery or will require another fast to allow the process of healing to continue. The earlier that corrective therapy is employed, the greater the chance of a lasting recovery.

Fasting and natural diet, though essentially unknown as a therapy, should be the first treatment when someone discovers that he or she has a medical problem. It should not be applied only to the most advanced cases, as is present practice.

Beth was a severe asthmatic and had a history of recurrent hospitalizations before she came under my care. At first we avoided further hospitalization only by keeping her on high doses of inhaled steroids, as well as other medication. Frequently, we had to add oral steroids in addition to the inhaled steroids when her condition took a turn for the worse. She was never in good control of her asthma even with high doses of medication and always endured wheezing and poor air flow. She awoke nightly to use her breathing machines.

Although she followed a careful diet, we saw no improvement. We talked about fasting, but she was not able to set a definite date to begin a fast because of her work responsibilities and her fear of undertaking a prolonged fast. I encouraged her to speak with some patients who were fasting and to observe firsthand how comfortable they were, and to speak to other patients who had undertaken long fasts to ask about their experiences. She took my advice, and after seeing patients fasting in comfort and talking with them about their experiences, she decided to fast. But it took her an additional two years of suffering with her severe asthma before she finally was able to get the time off from work and to gather the courage to begin.

Slowly, through the first week of the fast, as Beth's breathing improved, we tapered her medication. Within four days of beginning the fast she developed a red, itchy rash all over her arms and legs. This represented the elimination of retained toxins that her body had never effectively been able to remove while she was eating and taking medication, especially because she was habitually on steroids. I assured her that this type of rash is extremely common in patients who have been on steroids in the past, because these medications suppress the body's self-cleansing and detoxification mechanisms, permitting the retention of tissue waste products.

Taking an oatmeal bath a few times daily helped relieve her itching. The rash began to clear, her breathing improved, and by the eighth day of the fast we were able to safely stop all medications. Beth continued her fast for 21 days, and for the first time in years was on no medication or inhalers. I was unsure whether or not she still had a touch of asthma left; her peak flow measurements (a measure of expiratory air flow measured by a hand-held device that the patient breathes into as forcefully as possible) were still slightly below normal, and I suspected that, in such a severe case, she should undertake another fast six months after the first one to make sure her body had adequately normalized and healed.

Beth checked in with me at a follow-up visit a month later and informed me she still had a touch of asthmatic symptoms, though not requiring regular medication or steroids as in the past. Five months later she reported that this was the best year of her life, that she was exercising, sleeping well, and could finally live a normal life. With the encouraging results obtained so far, Beth is enthusiastic about getting completely well and excited about her positive experience with fasting. She is already planning her second fast. Often, patients like Beth, who once had a fear of the fast, become enthusiastic about the powerful healing properties of fasting and encourage others with similar problems to utilize this conservative, natural approach.

The Painful Symptoms of Inflammation Can Stop Without Drugs

Many recurrent and painful conditions besides asthma are the result of localized inflammation. The inflammatory process often causes painful symptoms that are not sufficiently understood by either physicians or lay persons. People are given drugs to cover up the pain of the inflammatory response, or are given anti-inflammatory medications to lessen it. But because the treatments do not remove the cause of the inflammation, they most often give only a temporary reprieve and a chronic condition results. After treatment with medications, it is not uncommon for individuals to experience gradual improvement of one inflammatory reaction, only to find that a new reaction has manifested itself elsewhere in the body.

Too frequently patients suffer from lifelong problems that are merely the response of irritated tissues to noxious stimuli. If the body had been given the chance to remove the noxious irritants, the troublesome chronic condition would never have resulted.

It is accurate to view inflammation as a corrective attempt by the body to restore normalcy to its cells and tissues. The inflammatory process is closely intertwined with the process of repair. Inflammation serves to destroy, dilute, or wall off the injurious agent. It is the reaction of living tissue to local injury. A series of events are set in motion by the body that attempt to heal and repair the damaged or threatened tissues. The inflammatory reaction calls the immune system into action, including entrapment of the irritants by specialized cells that attempt to ingest and neutralize the irritant. Fluid and blood cells accumulate in the area to dilute and destroy the injurious agent. If inflammation is not eventually resolved, and if the initiating causes are not eventually removed, further damage to the tissues may result.

Without inflammation, infections would go unchecked and wounds would never heal. Damage to our tissues and organs would ensue and cancer would be more likely to occur if the body did not diligently attempt to remove toxic substances from its tissues. It is common to think of bacteria or other microbes as the cause of inflammation, but almost all other causes of cell injury also provoke inflammation.

Fasting is an effective way to treat inflammation because it allows the body to remove the noxious stimuli that caused the problem in the first place. Rather than suppress the inflammatory response with steroids in the form of pills or inhalants, as is done in asthmatics, these medications are tapered off just prior to or even during the fast; then the body is able to resolve the inflammatory process while fasting so that it can accomplish the remedial act of removing the noxious causes of the inflammation.

When we view the inflammation as the problem and not the result of the problem, we make an essential error in health care. The result is that doctors wind up treating symptoms rather than causes, and the patient becomes forever cursed to a lifetime of disease and medical treatments.

Frequently the typical physician searches for an infectious agent that may be causing the painful symptoms and finds none. He then may become frustrated when he cannot find something to treat or kill with drugs, his only weapon. His only recourse is to give pain medication or anti-inflammatory drugs, not knowing what he is treating. This well-meaning physician is treating the inflammatory response, which is not the cause of the illness. He is trying to suppress the efforts of the body to remove poisonous waste. Remember, the inflammatory response itself is trying to protect you. The body does what it must in its attempt to protect your long-term health.

If, instead of taking drugs, a gentle diet of only fresh fruits and raw vegetables is consumed for a few days, and, if needed, a short fast is undertaken, the body would be able to complete the repair process, remove the retained waste or other toxin, and restore its tissues to normal.

Instead, the body is almost never allowed to complete its repair work. The individual never reflects on his or her stressful dietary and life-style practices, and the doctor does not consider these as possible culprits. This is why I see patients with a multitude of various inflammatory conditions that have never resolved. In fact, one could list hundreds of various ailments that are difficult to treat by modern medicine, but respond predictably to an approach that emphasizes and respects the power of the body to restore itself to normalcy by removing the impediments to healing.

Fasting to Lose Weight Without Changing Your Diet Is Pointless

Since about 70 percent of our population is overweight, why isn't an entire chapter of this book devoted to obesity? Many books about fasting focus predominately on weight loss. The answer is that while most of the patients whom I fast are indeed overweight, they usually have some underlying medical condition in addition to being overweight that brought them to the fast. They fast and they do lose weight, but most of them follow my dietary recommendations first, before the fast, often losing 50 pounds or more as a result of their new style of eating before the fast even begins. I usually have my patients take off the "easy-to-lose" weight first, and then have them fast, to help them achieve a really healthy and lean body.

If a person is unable or unwilling to make permanent changes in the diet and to follow a healthy eating plan before and after the fast, there really is no point in fasting. If people are concerned with losing weight, they must make permanent life-style and diet changes that they are willing to live with for the rest of their lives.

Diets don't work, because no matter how much weight you lose on a diet, when you go off it the weight will come back again. Likewise, if individuals fast and then go back to their former ways of eating, they will eventually regain all the weight and the benefits of the fast will be wasted. Therefore, I do not generally encourage my overweight patients to fast. It is more important for them to adopt a healthy diet and life-style to maintain their health and prevent disease. A slim, healthy body will then occur naturally as a consequence of their new habits, which include better food and, of course, regular exercise.

Later, after losing most of the excess weight, if someone wants to fast to drop the last 20 to 40 pounds that are so difficult to lose, I encourage it, because the person has already shown his or her ability to stay with a healthy diet, and I know the results of the fast will further encourage the person never to go back to the former way of eating. If the individual stays on a natural food, vegetarian diet after the fast, he or she will not regain weight. In fact, those who experience the rejuvenating effects of the fast look slimmer and feel younger and healthier than they have since they were kids.

One must be warned, however, that fasting slows down the metabolism, and that this lowered metabolic rate can last for four to six weeks after the fast. One must eat very carefully and not overeat or go off the prescribed diet during this period after the fast. A few pounds of weight will usually return in the next week or two after breaking the fast as the body replenishes the fluid and electrolytes that it lost while fasting.

When I fasted, my taste, hearing, and eyesight all improved. I also routinely hear this reported by others who fast. Because of this improvement in the ability to taste, simple natural foods taste better. I remember eating that first piece of lettuce after a fast and remarking that I never realized that lettuce tasted sweet before. After I arrived home from my fast in Texas, I soon went to try a taste of peanut butter, because that was one of my favorite foods in the past. I put a small spoonful of a popular brand of peanut butter into my mouth, but had to quickly spit it out and rinse the horrible taste from my mouth. My taste buds had changed so much from fasting and become so much more sensitive that the peanut butter tasted like a mouthful of heavily salted chemicals.

You Can Win at Weight Loss

Many of you know that the conventional answer to being overweight—low-calorie dieting—is not an effective solution to the problem. For the vast majority of people, being overweight is not caused by how much they eat, but by *what* they eat. It is a myth that people get heavy because they consume too many calories.

When researchers compare overweight and thin people, they find that both groups consume roughly the same amount of calories.[6,7,8] What makes overweight people different is the amount of fat they eat. The facts are that as long as you are eating fatty foods you won't be able to lose weight.

The food our bodies need more than any other is carbohydrate. Our muscle cells and brains are designed to run on the glucose derived from carbohydrate. We need 35 times more carbohydrate than protein for growth and 800 times more carbohydrate than fat. For example, an adult human requires about 20 grams of protein a day to maintain cell replacement and repair, about 700 grams of carbohydrate, and about 3 grams of fat. The average American consumes, daily, about 150 grams of protein—8 times the actual need—and often more than 100 grams of fat.

If your diet is deficient in carbohydrate, you will have to consume a great deal more in an attempt to feel satisfied. Along with that intake of food will come huge quantities of fat if you are eating the typical American diet or are following many other weight-loss plans. The effect is that you'll be overweight, your hunger won't be satisfied, and you'll crave sweets.

Not so long ago, many people believed that complex carbohydrates were fattening. Dieters would avoid starchy foods such as potatoes, beans, and pasta. It turned out that the real culprits were the high-calorie greasy toppings such as butter, sour cream, and high-fat salad dressings. Healthy foods such as vegetables, whole grains, and fruits contain adequate protein and are rich in carbohydrate, but have little fat.

If you wish to commit suicide with food, killing yourself as quickly as possible with a heart attack, cancer, or stroke, focus your diet on fat-based foods such as meats, most dairy products, vegetable oils, and salad dressings rather than on fruits and vegetables—the complex carbohydrates. Fats are the bad guys; carbohydrates are the good guys.

If the body tries to store the energy from carbohydrates it must first convert it to fat, a process that in itself consumes 23 percent of the consumed calories. In contrast, if you eat fat, and the American diet holds about 40 percent of its calories from fat, your body stores it as fat with only 3 percent of its calories burned in the process. This is why calories from fat are more likely to increase body fat than the same number of calories from carbohydrate. To make matters worse, fats in the diet slow down your metabolic rate. In contrast, carbohydrates speed it up.

The way to achieve permanent weight control and a long healthy life—free of the leading chronic diseases such as diabetes, heart disease, cancer, and osteoporosis—is to base your diet on grains, beans, vegetables, and fruits. These are the most powerful foods for controlling weight, and most people can eat all they want of them and stay slim and healthy.

What is wrong with every single commercial weight-loss program? They are all too high in fat because they cater to the American love affair with rich, high-fat food. Weight Watchers brand foods contain 24 percent of calories from fat. Lean Cuisine contains 25 percent of calories from fat. All commercial diet plans, since they are not very low in fat, must restrict portion sizes to offer "low-calorie" meals.

You may be able to take fewer breaths per minute for a few minutes, but in about an hour or so you will be hungry for air and will be forced to speed up your respiratory rate. In the same way, it is merely a matter of time before someone on one of these diets, trying to keep portions small, will again increase the amount of food he or she consumes. When this happens, the weight will return with a vengeance.

Ninety-nine percent of all people who lose weight on a diet gain it back again.[9] This incredibly high failure rate holds true for all weight-loss schemes, programs, and diets. Fasting merely to lose weight, and not coupled with the nutritional guidelines contained in this book, would likewise be a failure for the same reason.

All the diet plans fail because people can't be expected to stay hungry and control their portion sizes forever. The urge to eat more food eventually becomes too great, so the weight is regained. You can't eat out of boxes and consume powdered drinks forever, so though you may lose some weight, you will always gain it right back. Instead, permanent changes in your eating habits must be made. Learning new recipes and different ways to eat will enable you to maintain your weight loss and your health.

If you desire to lose weight effortlessly, adopt a diet that primarily consists of fresh fruits, vegetables, whole grains, and beans. This is a diet with less than 10 percent of calories from fat. I can assure you that the fat will effortlessly melt away from your body.

When diets attempt to keep your caloric intake very low, your body slows down its metabolic rate because it senses the need to conserve fuel. The more your food intake drops, the harder your body will try to keep from losing its fat. The effect is significant. On a 500-calorie diet your metabolic rate can drop 20 percent below normal. This reaction is frustrating to dieters, who often find that the longer they diet, the harder it becomes to lose weight.

The unfortunate result of denying oneself food as a means of diet control is that when the dieter goes back to eating normally, fat more easily accumulates because of a low metabolic rate. This leads to the familiar yo-yo phenomenon in which dieters lose some weight, only to rebound to a heavier weight than they started with.

In contrast, I tell my patients to eat as much food as they can. In fact, when they are eating foods that are rich in water-soluble fiber but contain less than 10 percent of calories from fat, they can stuff themselves and still enjoy substantial weight loss.

Oils are 100 percent fat. No matter what the type, oil is 100 percent fat. Like all other forms of fat, it contains 9 calories per gram. Carbohydrates hold only 4 calories per gram. That means oil contains more than twice the calories of carbohydrates.

When we put concentrated fat in our diet, the body easily converts it to body fat. This is more important than the total number of calories we consume.

How many baked potatoes do you think you can eat to get the same amount of fat as in 1 teaspoon of olive oil? If you said 70, you are right. Which do you think will make you feel more satisfied, one teaspoon of oil or 70 baked potatoes?

Some Weight-Loss Schemes Are Dangerous

Advertisements and claims about weight-loss plans and products that aid weight loss bombard us daily. There are countless ways to lose weight, but besides the false claims and rebound weight gain that come with all these diet schemes, many of them are not safe.

For example, one way to control your weight is to smoke cigarettes, especially if you snort cocaine at the same time. Don't laugh. Some people really do this. Thank goodness most of us know this will put us at significant risk of heart attack and sudden death, so it is not our weight-loss program of choice.

Another example of a dangerous way to lose weight is to follow a high-protein, carbohydrate-restricted diet. Yet despite their proven dangers, these diets are still suggested by some physicians.

Weight loss can occur on a high-protein, low-carbohydrate diet in a way similar to how sick cancer patients lose weight or diabetics lose weight when their blood sugar levels get too high. When the body can't find enough carbohydrate to properly run its machinery, it looks for emergency fuel that can be utilized in times of crisis, fasting, or starvation. This fuel is called **ketones.** Ketones are a fat breakdown product that many cells can use as an alternative (emergency) fuel rather than carbohydrate. As ketone production increases a condition called ketosis occurs and the acids rise in our bloodstream. This can be measured by checking the acidity of our urine.

If the dieter maintains a high-protein, low-carbohydrate program for a prolonged period of time, the excess protein consumed that cannot be stored in the body, as well as all the acids created by protein metabolism and as a result of ketosis, must be eliminated by the kidneys. As a consequence the kidneys become overworked and enlarged. Kidney damage will slowly occur. This is in contrast to fasting ketosis because during fasting, no excess protein by-products are excreted, only a mild acidosis occurs, and the fasting condition is maintained for only a short duration.

Those individuals who follow high-protein weight-loss plans inevitably speed up the aging of their kidneys and unknowingly destroy functional units in the kidneys called **nephrons.** It often takes years for this damage to be detected by blood tests. By the time it is detected, irreparable damage might have already been done, because the signs that damage has occurred will not be noticeable by blood test until more than 80 percent of the kidneys are destroyed. This can be especially dangerous in diabetics or individuals with high blood pressure because their kidneys are already under stress from their medical condition.

Additionally, as these acids are washed through the kidneys, many minerals (especially calcium) stored in the bones are washed out too. Osteoporosis very frequently occurs in people who follow this type of weight-loss plan for prolonged periods. That is, if they live long enough, because it is well established that a diet with a high proportion of animal foods increases our risk of premature death from every leading cause.

Every single person who follows a high-protein, carbohydrate-restricted diet will speed up the aging of the kidneys and increase the risk of kidney stones and nephrocalcinosis (hardening of the kidney). Even worse, since animal-based foods are almost 100 percent fat and protein, and contain no carbohydrate or fiber and none of the protective antioxidant nutrients, a diet based on animal food is closely linked to early death from cancer (especially colon cancer, prostate cancer, and breast cancer) and heart attack.

Liquid protein diets, or protein-modified fasts, have caused the death of more than 60 people.[10,11] Certainly Americans soon will realize that you can't purchase health in a can or bottle.

Don't be conned into a quick way to get something for nothing. You can't poison your body with toxic drugs and expect not to reap the consequences down the road. Likewise, you can't poison your body with an unhealthy high-fat or high-protein diet and expect not to pay the price with the eventual deterioration of your health.

Other Conditions Respond to Therapeutic Fasting

Nature tells us to fast. When we have no appetite during an acute illness, fasting is nature's way to accelerate recovery. Feeding the sick individual when his digestive powers are diminished and weak only serves to further complicate the illness. In an acute viral illness, fasting activates white blood cells and causes more interferon to be produced.

When animals other than humans feel sick, they do not eat. Listen to your body when you are sick and have no appetite. Fast for a few days, then proceed to a light diet of fruit and salad vegetables for a few days and you will quickly recover your health. Your body will have used the viral attack as a friend to your future well-being and aided in nature's plan to give your system a quick internal housecleaning.

Diseases such as acne and eczema, tinnitus (chronic noise in the ears), vertigo, fibromyalgia, glaucoma, cervical dysplasia, chronic neck and back pain, polymyalgia rheumatica, and many others are helped by fasting. I have witnessed patients with severe hypothyroidism (not producing sufficient thyroid hormone) who have had their blood tests normalize after fasting. Even deafness has resolved during fasting for some other condition, surprising both the patient and the doctor when the hearing returned.[12]

Fasting is also useful for a variety of other chronic ailments because the beneficial effects of the fast are not disease specific. Physicians who have used this approach have recorded improvement or recovery from conditions of every description that patients had been needlessly suffering with for years. Besides the diseases already mentioned, one should assume that in the vast majority of chronic medical conditions this approach may give the disease sufferer the best chance to achieve a complete recovery and avoid a lifetime of suffering or medical treatments.

Sometimes when people try to make major dietary changes without the benefit of fasting they become frustrated. Beneficial changes that can take months or years with careful eating happen quickly if a fast is utilized. Once a person begins to realize the health potential and can see the results, he or she is more likely to become committed to a lifetime of healthful living.

The withdrawal symptoms of addiction to such drugs as alcohol, cocaine, nicotine, and caffeine are resolved quickly while fasting. Most people are amazed at how easy it is to quit smoking while fasting. Those who have fasted begin to respect their body in a new way that enables them to take better care of themselves in the future.

People often start getting the warning signs of chronic disease when they are young. Generally, they go to their physicians with frequent infections as children. As teenagers they develop acne and allergies, and often take drugs to suppress symptoms. Years later, they gradually become medically dependent, having to take medications for the rest of their lives. Fifty percent of our population over the age of 60 takes some medication.

If we teach our children from a young age that disease is not inevitable and not to be expected, and if we build good health into our lives, we will have a chance to have a healthy society.

This book illustrates and emphasizes a powerful philosophy, a revolutionary way of thinking about health and disease. It is not merely about fasting, it is about realizing that we have lifetime responsibility to maintain our health. If we protect our families and our children from the causes of ill health, we will prevent needless suffering in the future.

9 | A Chapter for Physicians and for Readers Who Want More Technical Information

Training in Fasting Supervision for Medical Doctors

Fasting is such a safe and effective modality for a variety of medical conditions that the supervision of this therapy should become routine for primary care physicians. Medical students have spent their monthly clinical rotations with me to learn more about this modality firsthand. Another month's rotation as an elective during residency would be an ideal way for physicians to become adequately trained.

In this chapter, I will discuss possible side effects and complications of fasting, assuming that the benefits of fasting were adequately reported in the other parts of this book. This is not intended to be a complete treatise for the medical professional on all aspects of caring for the fasting patient. It is merely an overview, discussing some of the major points of interest.

A residency-trained medical doctor, with knowledge of internal medicine and electrolyte imbalances, and with an adequate nutritional background, should be able to become appropriately skilled to conduct fasts after one week of lectures at a conference set up for such a purpose. Presently, there are numerous conferences available for physicians to attend to learn more about various nutritional interventions for chronic diseases. Interested physicians can contact me at the following address for more information about such training:

Joel Fuh'rman, M.D.
Amwell Health Center
450 Amwell Road
Belle Mead, New Jersey 08502
Telephone: (908) 359-1775
Fax: (908) 359-2068

The International Association of Professional Natural Hygienists

The IAPNH, an organization of primary care doctors specializing in the application of therapeutic fasting, offers certification for its members in fasting supervision. The members of this organization include licensed medical doctors, osteopaths, chiropractors, and naturopaths. Certification for fasting supervision does not occur unless the doctor has undergone at least a six-month approved residency with a certified professional to gain experience in therapeutic fasting.

A list of certified members of the IAPNH can be requested through their organization at:

IAPNH c/o Attorney Mark Huberman
204 Stambaugh Building
Youngstown, Ohio 44503

The Necessity of Physician Supervision

Fasting is such a safe therapeutic intervention that many laypeople argue that daily supervision by a physician is not necessary. Although it is true that fasting is both natural and safe, all prolonged fasts **must** be supervised by a physician with expertise and knowledge. Fasting longer than two to three days should not be undertaken by patients on their own. It is important for a physician to dissuade a person who wants to undertake a prolonged fast without proper supervision.

A physician must monitor the fast to guarantee the safety of the patient. It is important to make sure the fast is terminated before an individual begins to develop low levels of electrolytes or other essential nutrients. Most patients can fast safely for 30 days or more. It is rare, but others, even after 10 to 15 days of fasting, may develop low levels of potassium and have to terminate the fast.

A trained physician should be able to distinguish a typical side effect or detoxification symptom of a fast from harmful symptoms that indicate the fast should be broken or that a blood test should be quickly run to make sure the fast is safe to continue. For example, a symptom such as dramatically increased weakness accompanied by a drop in blood pressure usually indicates the fast should not continue.

A similar situation occurs during childbirth. Most people understand that childbirth is a relatively safe and natural process. Occasionally, however, intervention by a trained professional is needed to optimize the outcome when signs might indicate a problem. The same is true for fasting.

It is reasonable for an otherwise healthy individual to fast for two or three days without medical supervision when suffering from an acute illness and decreased appetite. This commonly occurs. Even then, if unusual symptoms develop, such as vomiting, and there is the possibility of dehydration, medical intervention should be sought immediately.

The Biochemistry of Fasting

Fasting is not starvation, and the terms should not be used interchangeably. The fasting period represents the time one can safely abstain from food and typically varies among individuals, based on tissue reserves and body weight. When a person abstains from all food and drink except water, the body utilizes nonessential tissues such as adipose tissue, digestive enzymes, and muscle tissue for fuel. Only when fasting is sustained and the nonessential tissue stores become inadequate to fuel the metabolic needs of the body does the body begin to metabolize essential tissues (e.g., vital organs) and starvation occurs. Even a thin individual has sufficient reserves to fast for approximately 40 days and not experience symptoms of starvation.

Weight loss is most rapid early in the fast. On the average, fasters lose approximately 1 pound per day. They may lose 2 pounds or more per day early in the fast but this rate drops off to about a half a pound daily later on, so the average weight loss usually remains at 1 pound daily. Fasters lose more weight if they are overweight; thinner individuals lose less weight. The early fasting-induced diuresis (water loss) causes an increased initial weight loss from the increase in urinary excretion of water and salt, but these 1 to 2 kilograms are regained rapidly with refeeding.

In fasting, the body undergoes a series of hormonal and metabolic changes to conserve its body mass and draw selectively from its supply of energy in adipose tissue, sparing the breakdown of muscle or enzymes. For each individual the ratio of fat to muscle tissue lost differs, dependent on initial body conditions, especially the amount of body fat.

Early in the fast, glycogen reserves in the liver are broken down to maintain glucose levels. The liver stores only about 100 to 125 grams of glucose as glycogen, however, and this stored glucose is rapidly depleted, usually in the first day of the fast.

When the fast progresses beyond the depletion of these glycogen reserves, the body muscles and internal organs (e.g., the liver and heart) obtain their energy predominantly from fatty acids derived from adipose tissue. However, fatty acids cannot supply all our energy needs. Small amounts of glucose are still needed to fuel the brain and red blood cells, which do not have the ability to be fueled by fatty acids. During the fast, the brain demands almost 80 percent of the rested body's fuel requirements, about 180 grams of glucose per day, and must continually receive an adequate supply.

From day 2 onward, the body manufactures the needed glucose through two metabolic pathways. The first source is glycerol derived from adipose tissue. However, the fat-triglyceride-glycerol-glucose pathway alone cannot produce sufficient quantities of glucose once the liver stores of glycogen are depleted. Thus a second, predominant source of glucose is obtained from the catabolism of muscle tissue. Some muscle loss is obligatory as the body utilizes amino acids from muscle tissues to synthesize glucose.

The fasting individual would need to catabolize over a pound of muscle mass a day to meet his or her glucose requirements. By the third day of the fast, however, the liver begins generating large quantities of ketones. As the level of ketones rises in the bloodstream they compete with glucose as a substance that can be used for energy in the central nervous system, thereby greatly diminishing the body's need for glucose, sparing protein, and preventing further acidosis caused by tissue catabolism. Through this inherent survival mechanism, the brain, muscle, and heart begin to use ketones instead of glucose as fuel. Muscle wasting at this time decreases to less than 0.2 kg per day. This is known as **protein sparing.** In this phase, muscle is conserved and the maximum breakdown of fatty tissue and removal of atheromas and toxins occur.

Ketosis develops within 48 hours in fasting females and 72 hours in males. However, ketosis in the fasting individual differs from that in diabetics. In uncontrolled diabetics, the levels of ketones produced reaches such high levels that the acid/base balance may be overwhelmed. In the fasting individual, the body maintains control of the levels of ketones produced as a fuel source.[1,2]

The unique nutritional adjustments that occur during a total fast, including the adaptation to ketone nutrition, apparently have long-term beneficial effects on brain function, improving psychological health as well as physical well-being. When EEG (electroencephalogram) data and endocrine parameters are measured during and after fasting, it appears the homeostasis mechanism of the body significantly improves in the central nervous system.[3]

Fasting Supervision and Contraindications to Fasting

It is the job of a trained physician to be able to distinguish those patients who are proper candidates for fasting from those who are not. It cannot be assumed that every individual can fast safely for a prolonged period of time—or at all. Occasionally it is necessary to end the fast many days before the patient wants to or the doctor intended to.

A physician should evaluate the patient on a daily basis. He must monitor blood pressure, pulse, and any other parameter that may be appropriate for that individual. Blood tests should be monitored at least weekly to assure adequate electrolyte balance and reserve as well as to check hydration status. With the appearance of sudden weakness or persistent vomiting, additional laboratory work is appropriate to assess electrolytes and hydration status.

Rarely, a patient may be encountered who cannot fast. For instance, some people have an enzyme defect called MCAD (medium-chain acyl-CoA dehydrogenase) deficiency, and it would be unsafe for these individuals to fast. MCAD is one of the enzymes needed for the oxidation of fatty acids. A deficiency in this enzyme is one of the most common inborn errors of metabolism. Since fatty acid oxidation is required as an alternate energy source during fasting, this disorder may go undiagnosed until a person attempts to fast. Even though this condition is exceedingly rare, respiratory failure, extreme weakness, seizures, coma, or death may ensue if the individual continues with a prolonged fast. This disorder is recognized by vomiting or extreme lethargy early in the fast; in addition, the urine does not show ketones as in a normal person who undergoes food deprivation.

Proper supervision also involves a blood test prior to the fast to ensure adequate liver and kidney function. I do not recommend fasting for patients with laboratory findings of significant liver or kidney disease. Extremely weak and debilitated patients generally should not fast. Nor should patients with severe anemia, severe nutritional deficiency states, porphyria, or pregnancy. Patients who are severely malnourished, such as those with advance stages of cancer or AIDS, should not fast because fasting will likely contribute to their malnourished state and perhaps to an earlier death.

Generally, medications should be tapered and discontinued prior to the fast whenever possible. Normally, I taper medication as the patient adopts a healthy diet and postpone the fast until it is safe to discontinue most medication.

Frequently, I encounter patients taking multiple chemotherapeutic agents, such as oral gold and methotrexate, who desire to fast. I do not fast these patients until they can be stabilized with less toxic medication. This is because of my concern that certain drugs when combined with fasting can potentially cause toxic insult to the kidneys. If these patients cannot reduce their dependency on such agents through appropriate dietary and nutritional management prior to the fast, they are not desirable candidates for a fast.

Clearly, a list can be made of hundreds of medications that should not be combined with therapeutic fasting. It would be inappropriate to compile such a list here. Suffice it to say that, except in rare instances, a patient should be stable enough to be able to stop all medication either before a fast or within a few days after the fast has begun, or a fast should not be entertained.

Extreme caution is necessary when fasting a person who has taken oral steroids for a prolonged period in the recent past. Even if the individual has been slowly weaned off the drug well in advance of the fast, adrenal gland suppression is still possible. As a result, fasting could cause an excessive loss of sodium, low blood volume, and rapid heart rate. These parameters should be more closely monitored in such patients. The fast may have to be discontinued at the onset of such signs or symptoms.

In cases in which hormone replacement is essential (for instance, with panhypopituitarism or hypothyroidism), administration of the appropriate hormone(s) may be continued during the fast. However, blood parameters should be observed and the medication dose lowered accordingly, because these patients generally require much less medication during the fast than when eating. Thyroid medication, for example, should be tapered to about one half the patient's usual dose a few days prior to the fast and then periodically monitored with blood tests to ensure the correct dose is being given.

Patients taking drugs such as antidepressants, tranquilizers, or narcotics should not fast. Patients on anticoagulation therapy with Coumadin or chemotherapeutic agents should not fast. Aspirin and other NSAIDs should be discontinued prior to the fast because of the increased risk of gastric irritation during the fast.

Oral hypoglycemics must be discontinued prior to the fast and insulin should be tapered off in the type II diabetic. Type I diabetics should not undergo a prolonged fast.

Since fasting is so effective at lowering blood pressure, hypertensive medication should be stopped prior to or early in the fast. For patients with dangerously high blood pressure who require some medication in the early stages of the fast, a transdermal clonidine patch is usually tolerated well. The patch is needed only temporarily, until blood pressure decreases to a satisfactory level. Nitrates are compatible with fasting as long as the blood pressure is not too low, and can be continued in patients with angina. Angina, however, invariably resolves with fasting, thereby eliminating the need for nitrates at some point in the fast.

Breaking the Fast

It is very important that the reintroduction of food after an extended fast begin very gradually. The body needs a period of time to stimulate the production of digestive enzymes that has been temporarily stopped by the fast. The fast is typically broken on one half of an orange or a piece of watermelon the size of a woman's fist every two hours on the first day. Over the next three days, the amount of food given is gradually increased and the interval between feedings is lengthened, so that by day 4 the person is able to comfortably tolerate three normal-size meals.

The foods eaten during this period are fresh fruits, lettuce, steamed vegetables such as zucchini and asparagus, and baked squash or sweet potato. Other physicians who employ fasting in their practice often break the fast with fresh fruit and vegetable juice and then gradually introduce food. My reasoning for usually breaking the fast on whole food is to begin to provide some bulk to encourage peristalsis, thereby encouraging the first bowel movement to occur before the patient leaves for home.

The stomach is very sensitive after the fast so one must be very careful not to break the fast on fruit that may be too ripe. For example, if an overly ripe, partially fermented pineapple is eaten, stomach cramping and pain may develop. Overeating too early after the fast may also result in abdominal pain and vomiting. Spicy food, and condiments such as salt and pepper, taken soon after fasting could irritate and cause damage to the stomach lining because the normal mucosal defense barrier has been diminished by fasting and takes time to return to normal.

Typical Signs and Symptoms of the Fast

Most of the symptoms experienced on the fast are mild and harmless and require no intervention other than reassurance and encouragement. However, other symptoms that may occur later during a prolonged fast may be signs of electrolyte insufficiency or other complications that would indicate the need to terminate the fast.

Blood pressure gradually decreases during the fast for numerous reasons, as discussed in Chapter 5. Fasting is also mildly dehydrating. Due to the possibility of orthostatic hypotension, which is falling blood pressure upon standing, the chief risk or side effect of prolonged fasting is the chance of fainting and injury sustained in the fall. The reason I have never had a patient faint during a fast I supervised is because I give appropriate warnings of this possible side effect and instructions to be careful. My patients are told not to jump out of bed quickly. All fasters are also instructed to get off their feet and lie down immediately if they begin to feel light-headed at any time. Men are told to sit down to urinate, especially when rising to do so in the middle of the night.

Occasionally, blood pressure falls to what could be considered very low levels. If this drop is pronounced and sudden, the fast should be broken. However, if the patient is otherwise stable and the exceedingly low blood pressure has been reached gradually from a relatively low pressure at the start of the fast, it should not be of concern. In addition, I have noted that a narrowing of the pulse pressure typically occurs when fasting. For instance, a reading of 80 over 70 is not unusual, especially for a person who did not have high blood pressure to begin with.

The pulse generally falls somewhat when fasting, reflecting the decreased workload of the heart. Any sudden change in vital signs, such as a sudden drop or rise in pulse, should be further evaluated by the physician to ascertain its benign nature, or the fast should be ended.

The hormonal changes that occur as the body attempts to conserve fuel on a prolonged fast frequently cause patients to feel colder than usual, and extra bedding is appropriate. I advise patients not to become too chilled or too hot as this wastes energy. I advise against sunbathing as the fast is already dehydrating, and the addition of sunbathing in hot weather may result in excessive and potentially dangerous dehydration.

Physiologic Side Effects of the Fast

In a patient with a history of atrial fibrillation, the early rise in ketoacids and the reduction in serum bicarbonate produce a mild but compensated metabolic acidosis. This mild acidosis can precipitate a return to an irregular rhythm. This typically reverts back to normal with refeeding or giving juice to such a patient. I terminate the fast if the patient does not remain in normal sinus rhythm. Patients with a history of sustained ventricular tachycardia (a life-threatening, heart rate irregularity) should not fast. In patients I have fasted who have had frequent ectopic beats, the ectopy has either improved or remained unchanged. If ectopy or abnormal ventricular complexes appear suddenly late in the fast, the fast should be broken immediately. This could indicate electrolyte imbalance or that the fast has been continued too long and starvation has begun. Occasional premature ventricular contractions may appear in the first few days of fasting; however, these typically resolve as the fast continues.

Patients generally do not have bowel movements during a fast. A typical patient fasting 10 to 30 days usually has one or none, until refeeding starts. There is the occasional risk that the first bowel movement after the fast may be hard and require a lubricant or suppository for comfort. I typically prepare the patients' bowel for the fast by having them eat primarily raw fruits and vegetables for a few days prior to the fast, which helps prevent difficulty with the first bowel movement afterwards.

If there is a history of constipation or sluggish bowel, it would be advisable to give a warm water enema during the first or second day of a prolonged fast to cleanse the bowel; this will ensure that there is no difficulty with the first bowel movement after the fast is broken.

Obviously, patients with inflammatory bowel disease may have multiple loose bowel movements during the early part of a fast. The bowel movements gradually diminish and eventually stop as the bowel heals from the effects of the fast.

Vomiting is an early side effect that occurs during the first few days in about 5 to 10 percent of patients who fast. This typically resolves with continuation of the fast. If the vomiting continues or is accompanied by diarrhea, the patient should be observed and treated appropriately for dehydration. In rare instances, dehydration from vomiting on a fast induces further vomiting, and the patient is unable to hold down any fluid or food, making it impossible to break the fast and refeed. This would be an indication for intravenous rehydration followed by breaking the fast.

Headaches are occasionally experienced by fasters early in the first day or two of fasting. However, most patients with a history of severe headaches or migraines are excited to observe that their headaches end as the fast continues. These withdrawal headaches should not be medicated during the fast as the detoxifying effects of the fast should be allowed to continue unhindered. If the fast is followed by a natural plant-based diet, the headaches can be cured permanently, as explained in greater detail in Chapter 4.

Insomnia is often experienced by fasters, but this varies greatly among individuals. Generally, the need for sleep is greatly diminished when we are not active and when our digestive tract is not at work digesting food.

Vitamin Supplementation During a Fast

Vitamin deficiency attributed to fasting is exceedingly rare. It normally doesn't occur on fasts less than 45 days in length unless the individual was depleted at the onset of the fast.[4] Taking vitamins during a fast is unnecessary and can create unpleasant symptoms.

Many of the physicians who have fasted patients and reported their findings in the medical literature have given vitamins during the fast. However, there is no evidence that this in any way increases the safety of a fast. During a total fast the gastrointestinal tract is better not disturbed with vitamin supplementation.

Sufficient vitamins, minerals, and macronutrients are released in appropriate proportions from tissue stores during the fast. Other physicians than myself who have fasted thousands of patients do not find vitamins of any value during this period.[5] This is confirmed by the observations of other researchers, who noted that vitamin deficiency due to involuntary fasting was very rare among famished populations during World War II, and reported only problems from vitamin supplementation during fasting.[6]

The body's own vitamin reserve more than meets the body's requirements while on a moderate-length fast. It has been proposed that fasting increases the ability of tissues to absorb and utilize nutrients.[7] From my experience, it is clear that we need not worry about the issue of vitamins in a fast of moderate length. I have found that the results of blood tests for vitamin and mineral levels change little during the fast; tests are expensive and unnecessary.

Blood Tests During the Fast

For patients undergoing prolonged fasts, blood tests and urinalyses are performed at approximately weekly intervals. This is necessary to help the physician decide how long to continue the fast. Some changes in laboratory parameters are normal, such as an elevation of uric acid. Other abnormalities, however, could indicate the fast should be concluded. Sometimes, moderate abnormalities in the blood tests or the patient's clinical status necessitate more frequent monitoring of these laboratory parameters.

Fasting almost always elevates the patient's uric acid level, frequently to very high values, but this does not cause gout and should be of no concern. The elevated uric acid levels are due to the increased breakdown of purines as well as the decrease in their elimination in the kidneys.

Some investigators have warned against fasting patients with a history of gout due to their concern that fasting may precipitate an attack. I believe that these fears are usually unfounded. What I and other physicians regularly employing fasts have observed is that even patients with a prior history of gout do not usually have attacks of gout on their fast. It is true that uric acid levels in the blood always rise to high levels in the fasting patient. Even with extremely high levels of uric acid, however, I have never seen an attack of gout on a fast. Other investigators report similar findings.[8,9] Dr. Shelton, who reported conducting more than thirty thousand fasts, asserted that never once did he see gout develop in a fasting individual, in spite of high levels of uric acid.

This illustrates that an elevated uric acid level is not the only cause of gout. There are reports in the medical literature of patients with acute attacks of gouty arthritis who have normal serum uric acid levels;[10] this illustrates that hyperuricemia and gout are often separate phenomena. Some other mechanism may be involved in gout besides the uric acid elevation, or the biochemical changes that occur in the fasting state may mitigate against the formation of uric acid crystals in the joints. Amazingly, even with supersaturation (uric acid levels rising to 18), episodes of gout are generally not experienced. There is a report of fasting precipitating an attack of gout in a patient who had frequent prior attacks.[11] My opinion is that even patients with a history of gout can fast safely if they follow a low-purine, vegetarian diet for three to six months prior to the fast and lose weight before the fast. This will resolve the gout condition before the fast begins.

Hemoglobin levels usually rise slightly during a fast, reflecting the hemoconcentration that occurs with a fasting-induced diuresis. If the hemoglobin value is too high, especially when accompanied by a relatively high BUN (blood urea nitrogen) level and high urinary specific gravity, the patient usually is not drinking enough water and must increase his or her water consumption.

Due to the body's built-in survival mechanisms, the amount of water needed while fasting is minimal. The desire for fluid diminishes and may be nil in some fasters. To minimize side effects and assure the safety of all patients, however, fasters need to be encouraged to drink water to prevent dehydration. One quart of water per day is usually sufficient for most individuals, but some need to be encouraged to drink two or more quarts, depending on their laboratory parameters.

Dehydration does not generally occur in the overweight patient. Rather, it is seen more frequently in the thin patient. If considerable dehydration ensues, the patient should be fed. Because dehydration due to fasting is secondary to electrolyte depletion, it is possible that increasing the amount of water given the faster will not be sufficient to correct the abnormality. Therefore, if serious dehydration results, the fast should be broken with an appropriate food such as fresh orange juice, vegetable juice, or watermelon.

One of my patients with asthma, who had tried to fast with another physician in the past, claimed she vomited and became nauseated whenever she fasted. Therefore, she could not fast for longer than a few days. After fasting her a few days, as predicted, she developed vomiting and nausea. I then looked at her blood and urine and it showed she was dehydrated with hemoconcentration (increased red blood cell concentration) and an increased BUN level. When I asked her if she was drinking at least four glasses of water a day as I had recommended, she said she never likes to drink much when she fasts. She was drinking less than 8 ounces of water a day. As soon as I corrected this by increasing her fluid intake, the problem stopped and she was able to fast without difficulty.

It is to be expected that the glucose level will fall and remain at low levels during the fast, typically between 40 and 65, except in the type II diabetic patient, who may have a near normal or slightly elevated glucose level during the fast. If it is imperative for a person with type I diabetes to fast, glucose levels should be tested regularly and the insulin dose appropriately adjusted to the lowered needs of the fast.

Electrolytes such as potassium, sodium, and chloride are exceedingly stable during a fast. Even though early in the fast the body loses quite a bit of sodium and potassium, this excretion falls as the fast progresses. Generally, the electrolytes remain at low normal levels throughout the rest of the fast. If the potassium level drops to 3.2, the fast should be broken unless the physician supervising the fast chooses to monitor the blood test more frequently to make sure the level does not continue to drop. Obviously, once the level has reached 3.2, one should not wait a week to run the next potassium check if the patient continues the fast. I recommend ending a fast for any person who has a potassium level lower than 3.0.

At any sign of sudden, extreme weakness during a fast, the potassium level should be considered suspect and rechecked. However, gradual loss of energy or the slow development of weakness as the body attempts to conserve energy by decreased activity is normal during the fast and to be expected.

Liver enzymes occasionally increase early in the fast. As the fast continues, they slowly return to normal. I have noted the elevation of liver enzymes more frequently in patients with autoimmune illnesses, connective tissue disorders, and psoriasis; this may represent the contribution that inadequate liver function contributed to their underlying disease state. In the psoriasis patient, for example, and even in fibromyalgia patients, the return to normal liver function during the fast or soon after parallels the improvement in their skin disease or symptoms of muscle pain.

Due to the large demands on the liver for energy metabolism early in the fast, bilirubin levels rise initially and then fall gradually as the liver adapts to the fasting state.[12]

Cholesterol levels increase considerably in the fast, reflecting a breakdown of atheromatous material. As discussed in Chapter 5, the level of total cholesterol may double over the patient's baseline in an individual with a history of atherosclerotic plaque, whereas the patient without diseased arteries will not show such an increase in cholesterol. Both LDL and HDL levels increase, but I have noted that the sharp rise in cholesterol in cardiac patients is predominantly of the LDL type.

Other researchers have noted minimal increases in cholesterol levels and a more predominant increase in the HDL component. These conflicting findings may represent the increased level of activity encouraged or permitted by other researchers and the fact that juices may have been consumed.[13] I interpret the strikingly higher elevation of LDL cholesterol seen in my fasting patients with atherosclerosis as being due to the increased effectiveness of the total fast over "juice fasting" in breaking down atheromas. I also forbid vigorous exercise, permitting only gentle back-mobility movements, flexibility and joint-mobility exercises, and a little walking.

Many physicians who routinely monitor blood cholesterol levels in their office are not aware that an elevation of cholesterol occurs even when a patient fasts overnight for a blood test and then has it drawn late in the day rather than in the morning. Fasting lipid profiles should be drawn first thing in the morning to prevent this phenomenon from disturbing the results.

Physicians may also be confused and the patient disappointed and discouraged when the individual who started adhering to a strict, extremely low-fat, zero-cholesterol diet has an increase rather than a decrease in his or her cholesterol level. I have noted from monitoring the lipid profiles of many such patients that not only is it possible to observe a temporary rise in triglycerides during this adjustment phase, but also the total cholesterol may occasionally rise significantly. When this occurs, it is observed during the first two to six months after the dietary change; then these lipid levels begin to drop and show notable improvement later on. My patients are often warned not to be discouraged by the early tests, which do not yet represent their significant decreased risk.

Reports of Death During Improperly Supervised Fasts

It is very important not to fast patients beyond their capacity. One cannot simply rely on how much body fat a person has to decide how long to fast that person. Even obese individuals can develop signs of starvation while still overweight if their muscle reserves fall to dangerously low levels while their fat reserves are still adequate. This would occur only when the fast was excessively prolonged, and has been reported in such patients who have fasted for many months. Cardiac failure could occur in patients who no longer have skeletal muscle reserve and who continue to fast. For this reason, I do not ever recommend a fast of more than 50 days even for obese individuals who feel well and look as though they could fast safely for months.

An obese patient died after seven months of fasting,[14] which, rather than illustrating the dangers, illustrates the safety of a prolonged fast. It is hard to imagine that anyone could recommend to a person, no matter how obese, to fast this length of time. After the protein-sparing phase of the fast begins, the body still requires a small quantity of muscle reserves to maintain an adequate level of glucose and other nutrients. If severely obese individuals fast long enough, they may still be overweight, but because their body habitat was mostly fat, not muscle, they could exhaust their muscle reserves while still maintaining an illusion of having sufficient nutrient reserves in their tissues to continue fasting. This gives the false impression that it is safe for them to continue to fast for a very long period of time, when actually, after fasting this long, their muscle reserves are depleted.

The medical literature contains a few studies in which obese patients died during a fast, apparently from ventricular arrhythmias. If we look in detail at these cases, we can clearly see that the individuals were fasted improperly, using multiple drugs during the fast, and had heart failure or renal disease prior to the fast.[15,16] For example, in a study reported by Spencer, ventricular arrhythmias occurred in two patients, one weighing 330 pounds who fasted 56 days, and the other weighing 233 pounds who fasted 21 days. These patients drank unrestricted amounts of coffee, tea, and fruit juice during the fast and were given digoxin, diuretics, and anticoagulants. These were not total fasts, and might be more appropriately called a coffee and fruit juice feast. Regardless, one should never fast a patient on diuretics and heparin, both of which are dangerous during a fast. It is also an added risk to drink coffee while fasting. Cardiac stimulants such as caffeine, and theophylline should be avoided.

Offering Patients a Choice

Fasting should be viewed as a natural physiologic process to which the body eagerly adapts itself. For many disease states fasting provides an appropriate condition for the body to recuperate under its own intelligent direction. The innate wisdom of the human body is a remarkable thing and vividly appreciated as the body sets itself to healing under the conditions of the fasting state.

Fasting for health under competent supervision can be a pleasant and rewarding experience that sets a patient on a new road of superior health. By employing this therapy in their practice, primary care physicians can now offer patients an alternative to drugs and the surgeon's knife, and gain fulfillment from seeing remarkable improvement in the health of their patients. For other physicians the knowledge of this nutritional approach is imperative so that, when appropriate, they can make referrals to a colleague who specializes in this therapeutic modality.

Rather than starting patients on drugs for chronic diseases, now physicians can offer suitable patients a chance to recover their health through natural diet and fasting. If dietary considerations, including the aggressive nutritional approach described in this book, are not offered and discussed with patients initially, their doctors are selling them short. These physicians are not disclosing all the pertinent information that patients need to make informed decisions about their health condition.

Whether the patient has a cardiac condition, hypertension, autoimmune disease, fibroids, or asthma, he or she must be informed that fasting and natural plant-based diets are a viable alternative to conventional therapy, and an effective one. The time may come when not offering this substantially more effective nutritional approach will be considered malpractice.

10

What to Expect on Your First Fast

In a fast we can observe the body gleefully going about getting rid of the toxins and wastes accumulated for years with the greatest capability and intelligence, all on its own.

—DR. WILLIAM ESSER

Who Should Fast?

Almost everyone can fast. Both the chronically ill and those with acute illnesses, such as viral infections, can utilize the fast to accelerate recovery. Even healthy individuals may choose to fast periodically. I am convinced that periodic fasting will prolong life. I am not speaking of frequent short fasts, a day or two long, but of an internal cleaning of 10 to 15 days' duration every five to ten years. In the field of longevity research, nothing else has as much solid, scientific documentation to support it as fasting and a natural-food based diet.

If you are suffering from any chronic disease, fasting makes even more sense. Fasting should not be used only as a last resort. It should be employed as the first mode of treatment before a physician starts you on medication for almost any chronic condition. If one can fast early in the disease process before years of steroids and other toxic drugs complicate the condition, it will be much easier to get well.

It is exciting to watch what a fast can do, because the power of the body to heal itself is wonderful to observe. This is especially striking because, as a physician, I see almost no self-healing in patients treated conventionally. They either get worse or their symptoms are palliated with drugs, while their health gradually deteriorates. The fast allows for self-healing.

213

Fasting is really not that exciting when you do it. The vast majority of people feel not much different from when they were eating. Many people do not even feel significant hunger. When one does feel hunger toward the end of the first day, it disappears in the next day or two.

The usual response I see is, "I can't believe I can feel so strong and well when I haven't eaten for fifteen days." This is the norm. When I did my 46-day fast, the only real complaint I had was boredom. Of course, I felt weak toward the end of such a long fast and had to rest in bed most of the day, but I actually attended my college classes full-time and felt great during the first 10 days of my fast.

Humans have been fasting for more than 50,000 years, long before modern-day doctors began embracing a drug approach to treating disease. It's hard to understand how people developed such a misconception about and fear of fasting. Perhaps it is because many people feel so bad when they skip just one meal, that they expect to feel that much worse if they skip so many more. The reality is, when you don't eat for a longer period of time, the discomfort quickly subsides and you actually feel better and better.

It is true that many people, because of their rich diets, can suffer withdrawal symptoms from the effects of their self-abuse and poor dietary practices (as explained in Chapter 4). Some may get headaches or experience hunger cramps when they don't eat; but these symptoms always end rapidly during the fast. As soon as the body gets the idea it is really fasting, the person feels better quickly. These mild symptoms of hunger or a mild headache are found to be exceptionally rare after the first day and practically nonexistent after day 2 of the fast.

As rare as these are, when a person does have withdrawal symptoms early in the fast, it is good they are getting them. This shows how much they really needed to fast. People who are most in need of a fast for detoxification purposes are those who feel the most discomfort with not eating. This should not stop anyone from fasting. So often I hear, "Oh I could not fast, I feel so miserable even if I skip one meal!" or, "I could not fast, I am hypoglycemic and if I don't eat I feel like I would die." These are exactly the people who most need to fast. They need to clean out all the wastes in their bodies that are causing these symptoms. One good fast followed by a health-supporting diet will banish such recurrent complaints forever.

Almost no one in America knows the meaning of the word hunger. In this country we mistakenly call the withdrawal symptoms from our rich diet "hunger." Stomach cramping is not hunger; a headache is not hunger. When truly healthy individuals who have been on natural, plant-based diets and who have avoided the typical disease-causing American diet fast, they do not experience cramping in the stomach or any other abdominal symptoms. Nor do they experience headaches when they skip a few meals. True hunger is solely a mouth and throat sensation and it is felt in the same area as thirst. No discomfort accompanies it. In fact, it makes food more enjoyable when we eat when we are truly hungry.

Unfortunately, almost all Americans are so overfed and actually subclinically ill from the typical modern diet that they have never experienced true hunger in their life and probably never will. The reason people mistake withdrawal symptoms, such as abdominal cramping and headaches, for hunger is that they experience these symptoms long before the sensation of true hunger appears. Many individuals who fast report, after eating again, that they finally understand the feeling of real hunger. They report it is great to now know when there is a real physiological need for food and to be able to listen to their bodies.

In any case, all these symptoms related to the first few days of fasting, whether you call them hunger or not, will not trouble you during the fast. They fade away as the body produces more ketones early in the fast, and as you begin to enter this metabolic phase unique to fasting.

Please don't make the mistake of grouping any unusual practice that is "something like" fasting on pure water to the real thing. For instance, protein-sparing modified fasts are very dangerous.

Fasting while taking diuretics and caffeinated beverages is also dangerous. Don't confuse a dangerous, improperly conducted fast with one that is correctly monitored and properly concluded after a safe period of time.

Certainly one should not fast if one is afraid of it. Do not fast if you are in turmoil about whether to fast or undergo bypass surgery, for example. Wait a little bit, speak to other fasters, observe some patients fasting in person, and talk to them. You don't want to be fasting while you are under emotional stress. This stress will interfere with the healing process and you will not get the maximum benefit.

How Long Should I Fast?

How long should you fast? It is probably best to let a physician experienced with fasting decide this for you. Most individuals who are fasting for an existing medical condition should fast between 14 and 28 days to get a significant benefit from the fast. I usually recommend at least two weeks, because I have seen from experience that it is after the first week that the large health benefits begin to reveal themselves.

Depending on the nutritional reserves of the individual, I prefer to fast a person with a chronic ailment close to three weeks. Most people of normal weight should not fast much longer than that because we do not want them to become so thin that they have a long road back regaining their strength.

Most people want to get back to work and their families quickly after the fast. Taking more than a month out of their life for this purpose is difficult for most. However, if you have a significant medical condition and decide to fast, it is best not to set a time period in advance. Rather, take it one day at a time. With your help, the physician monitoring your fast can determine its optimal length.

It is exceptionally unusual for anyone who undergoes a supervised fast for three weeks or less to develop dangerously low electrolyte stores, as three weeks is a relatively short period of time. Of the last 100 patients I have fasted, only one person had too low a potassium level to safely continue the fast after two weeks. He was planning to fast 30 days. When I told him he had to break his fast and start eating again, he initially became upset. He had read numerous books on fasting, considered himself educated on the subject, and questioned my judgment. I needed to explain to him that the reason he was fasting under a physician's supervision was just for a rare occasion such as this. The ability to suspect and detect when a person's electrolyte reserves might be running low is exactly why fasts should be physician-supervised. This patient understood that we couldn't gamble with his health and let his potassium level dip below 3.0.

Occasionally, individuals fast under my supervision for longer than 21 days. I have conducted numerous 30-day fasts and a few even longer, but those were the exceptions. Dr. Shelton, who fasted more than thirty thousand people, routinely fasted individuals for 21 to 40 days. He reported his longest supervised fast was 90 days, but I would consider a fast of this length risky, even if the person appears to have enough tissue reserves.

If one wants to try a fast some weekend, it is easy to fast from breakfast on Friday, with bed rest most of Saturday and Sunday. A small fruit meal at dinnertime Sunday evening would break the fast. In this manner a weekend fast every once in a while would give the body a brief internal rest and cleaning, and still allow the person to get to work on Monday morning.

If those with a cold or flu fast on their own for a few days, or if a healthy individual wants to fast for two to three days, there should be no objection but, in general, people should not fast repeatedly without sufficient time to allow the body to rebuild its nutritional reserves. Even short fasts at frequent intervals, like two days a week or one week per month, are not advisable.

For those who desire to undertake a more lengthy fast, or who have a significant medical condition, physician supervision and guidance is important. The physician chosen should have knowledge and experience in the fasting field. There are many of us now, and more are being trained every day.

What Should I Do During the Fast?

During the fast one should drink at least 1 quart of pure water daily, and more if thirst demands. Chlorinated tap water should not be used. Most fasting establishments utilize distilled water for this purpose. I utilize distilled spring water because it is the purest water I can purchase and is totally free of chlorine.

Since fasting is mildly dehydrating I do not encourage sunbathing or hot baths during the fast. I do not want the individual to get too hot or too cold. Most fasters get cold more easily during the fast and need an extra blanket at night. They are encouraged to keep warm and not to become chilled because this wastes energy.

I give my fasters gentle stretching exercises to do to keep their backs flexible, and encourage them to walk around a little, but discourage any strenuous exercise. Occasionally fasters develop some lower back discomfort. At first I attributed this to spending so much time in bed. But because this occasional occurrence of lower back discomfort resolves as the person continues the fast, I realized it was likely related to a biochemical rather than to a structural problem. Many aches and pains that appear and then resolve during the fast illustrate the heightened detoxification and reparative activity made possible by the fasting state.

Many people require less sleep during the fast than they do normally. One should still rest sufficiently and relax at night in a quiet room. Rest in the dark if you are unable to sleep, and do not fret or be concerned if you don't sleep much when you are fasting. Each person is different; try to rest and sleep as much as you can, but if you can't sleep much, that is OK, too.

We want to give the body a complete rest so that it can devote its energies to healing. Arguments, business problems, and family problems should be avoided. This is a time for recuperation and the person should be resting and at peace physically and mentally. The faster should spend most of his or her time in bed either relaxing, sleeping, or doing gentle activities such as reading, writing, or listening to the radio.

Many fasters listen to tapes, watch videos, and read books on natural health and healing while they are fasting. They read a few more books on fasting or go over the ones they have already read. They utilize the time to reinforce their commitment to a healthy life-style. Many talk about and read natural food cookbooks, as they have a keener awareness of food and the importance of putting high-quality, natural food into their bodies. They become excited at the prospect of making new, plant-based recipes.

Breaking the Fast—Food Never Tasted So Good

Finally—what most fasters have been waiting for. Most fasters look forward to this day, although a few always want to continue, to make sure they have totally cleaned out their bodies. I reassure them that with proper eating, their health will continue to improve. With that, they look forward to their first meal. And what a meal it is! Although it is small, the taste is mighty. After not eating, one's taste buds are extremely sensitive.

Correctly breaking the fast is very important. Foods must be introduced slowly and certain foods should not be eaten soon after a lengthy fast. The digestive enzymes need adequate time to restore themselves after a period of quiescence. The body shuts down the production of digestive enzymes and we must give it the chance to adjust to food again.

After about three weeks, most of my patients break their fasts with gradual increments of fresh fruits or vegetables. They follow a precise eating plan carefully designed for them for about five to seven days before going home. They continue to eat conscientiously at home. If they have been chronically ill, they usually follow specific dietary instructions that they take with them when they leave. By the time they are ready to go home, they have had their first postfasting bowel movement and are usually feeling well enough to manage on their own.

Typically, juicy fruits are the ideal food to use to break a fast. For the first feeding, watermelon, about the size of a woman's fist, or one half of an orange is given every two hours. The fasters are instructed to eat slowly and chew the food very well. Either fresh-squeezed vegetable or fruit juice may also be used, about 6 to 8 ounces every two hours on the first day.

On the second day I usually continue the "fruit only" diet with one medium-sized piece of fruit or melon every three hours. On the third day, four meals are given. Lettuce is introduced with the fruit. On the fourth day after the fast, the patients resume their three-meals-a-day schedules, but the size of each meal is still smaller than the usual prefast amount. At this time foods such as zucchini, tomatoes, and cucumber are added. A small amount of cooked vegetables such as butternut squash or potato can also be added at this time. Most of those who just completed a fast are overjoyed with each new addition of food.

The stomach is very sensitive after a long fast. Therefore, individuals should not be given pineapple or any other food that may be fermented or possibly be under- or overripe immediately after a fast. Dried herbs or spices can also be irritating to the lining of the digestive tract and should not be added to foods. The protective layer of mucus lining the stomach has thinned with fasting and takes a little time to restore itself. If the food is slightly rotten (for example, a slightly overripe pineapple) it may irritate the stomach and cause severe abdominal cramping. Dry food such as a baked potato, grains, or dried fruit should not be eaten to break the fast. It is important to eat high-water-content food for ease of digestion at this time.

If the person has a weakened digestive capacity, such as in irritable bowel disease, it is preferable to start with something gentle on the bowel, like a small, green zucchini, steamed until just soft.

Whole fruit is used more frequently than juice to break the fast because eating the entire food, fiber and all, will encourage a bowel movement a little sooner. Since fasters have not moved their bowels for quite some time, it is reassuring to them to have a comfortable bowel movement before they head home. It might be more appropriate to break the fast on juice if the potassium level is getting a little too low and the physician wants to bring it up quickly.

If a patient is overweight and has a tendency to gain weight easily, he or she should eat very carefully after the fast. These individuals should eat only raw fruits and vegetables with the addition of some lightly steamed green vegetables until they check in with their physician again in two or three weeks after the fast. Since their metabolic rate is low for the first month after the fast, we emphasize raw food over cooked carbohydrates, as this will prevent possible weight gain during this postfast period.

What Are the Side Effects of Fasting?

Fasting has occasional side effects. Actually, it is incorrect to call them side effects because in most cases these minor discomforts are the work of the remarkable self-healing powers of the body and not the effects of ingesting toxic substances, as are the side effects of most drugs. When compared to the risks of taking drugs or undergoing a surgical procedure, fasting is indeed side-effect free.

The typical symptoms felt on a fast are those detoxification symptoms that occur as the body attempts to rid itself of unhealthy substances. For instance, after about six days of fasting, one patient with ulcerative colitis developed a cough. She admitted to having quit smoking a few years earlier. The body was finally addressing the damage to the lungs and was sloughing off dead cells and debris built up from the many years of smoking.

Still, coughs, as well as other unpleasant symptoms of fasting, are unusual. In the last 100 patients I have fasted only two coughed for a few days, and both of them were former smokers.

My wife, Lisa, undertook her first fast after she developed urinary discomfort. She had experienced recurrent urinary tract infections throughout college. After just two days of fasting, her symptoms subsided. Now, twelve years later, she has never once experienced another urinary tract infection.

Fasting so effectively lowers blood pressure that another side effect is light-headedness. A patient whose blood pressure changes rapidly, and is unaccustomed to such a low pressure, could become light-headed and even faint. This is probably the greatest risk of injury on the fast; that is, the risk of injuring oneself in a fall due to light-headedness.

Although becoming light-headed is a rare occurrence, one must be prepared. Never has a patient of mine fainted while fasting, probably because I explain the following precautions. My patients are warned not to jump up out of bed in the middle of the night; instead, I direct them to sit on the bed's edge for a minute first. If a man rises to urinate in the middle of the night, he should urinate sitting down. This is because a person doesn't suddenly faint; instead, he or she will first feel light-headed and then, in a few seconds, may faint. All my patients are instructed that if they ever feel light-headed while walking, they must lie down on the floor or ground immediately and not continue walking.

A white, coated tongue frequently occurs within a few days of fasting. This signifies the elimination of waste through the tongue. Often I encounter patients who are eliminating through their tongue (while eating), and they or their doctor, seeing a white, coated tongue, thinks they have a yeast infection; this is not the case. With decreased caloric intake and the increase of ketones in the bloodstream, the tongue develops this coating. Sometimes there is a sensation of dryness in the mouth, and the coating on the tongue is associated with bad breath or a bad taste. The faster can leave the tongue alone or wipe the coating off partially with a wet washcloth. This elimination process does not bother the fasters. In fact, they usually welcome it as an indication of how much waste they are eliminating.

About 1 out of 20 fasters develops episodes of nausea or vomiting while on the fast. These episodes usually occur only once or twice. They are more likely to develop in those who are not drinking enough water and are mildly dehydrated. All fasters must drink at least a quart of water daily whether they feel like it or not. If the vomiting is continuous and severe, the fast should be broken. This too is exceedingly rare.

Another interesting phenomenon of a fast is that the person's urine usually darkens and even becomes cloudy at times. The urine often clears somewhat as the fast continues. Bowel movements generally cease on the fast, or the faster will have only one at some point during the fast. During my own fast, I had only one bowel movement, which occurred on the thirty-sixth day. A bowel movement during the fast may be malodorous, but should happen only once.

Other possible detoxification reactions that may occasionally occur on a fast are itchy skin lasting for a few days, a light rash that clears as the fast continues, and rhinorrhea ("running" nose). Usually, the area of the body where problems were experienced in the past is the one that shows activity. For example, a person with chronic sinus problems will eliminate more mucus from the nose early in the fast, an asthmatic may cough up mucus, and a person with recurrent vaginal symptoms may develop a malodorous vaginal discharge.

Interestingly, patients having mild elevations of their liver function as indicated by their blood test prior to fasting frequently develop some toxic elimination through the skin during the fast. This itching or rash develops before the liver function tests finally begin to normalize.

Many doctors employing the fast for healing purposes have called these troubling symptom a "healing or fasting crisis." They have used this term to denote these symptoms as eliminative efforts of the body, made possible by the powerful detoxifying power of the fast. Patients usually are satisfied when experiencing these symptoms because it shows them that the body is busy throwing out its garbage.

For the vast majority of patients the fast is completely comfortable and they experience no troubling symptoms. Some patients complain that they are too comfortable. They were expecting to feel something out of the ordinary. I have been asked many times, "Am I getting well, because I don't feel bad enough to feel anything is happening?" I reassure them that they do not have to experience an eliminative reaction for the fast to be healing and detoxifying.

Remember, as you read about all the possible things you can feel on a fast, that all of these troubling symptoms are not typical. Rather than experiencing side effects, most fasters experience positive signs. Their aches and pains resolve; their smell, eyesight, and hearing improve; and after the fast their ability to taste dramatically improves. Even their emotions improve: they have less nervous irritability as the level of retained waste in their body is lowered.

When I fasted, a mole I had on my arm fell off. Benign skin lesions and other bumps such as subcutaneous lipomas often shrink and disappear if the fast is long enough.

A person's energy level is obviously lower during a fast. This is usually proportional to the amount of fat reserve. Heavy people lose more weight and have more energy on their fast. I have seen overweight individuals fast 30 days or more and have the same energy they did while eating. Thin people lose less weight and have less energy reserve available, so they eventually feel weaker on the fast. As the reserves of the body decrease, weakness occurs and the faster needs to rest more. Thin fasters should be encouraged to rest in bed much of the time to conserve their body weight.

What Happens After the Fast Is Broken?

After people undergo an extended fast, they are quite satisfied with the small amount of food served and sometimes feel full even when they don't finish the portion. One must be careful not to overeat at this time. If you think you are too thin, don't worry about it; if you take it slow, your digestion will be excellent now and you will be building muscles in no time. You now have the opportunity to rebuild your body with wholesome food. This is a rebirth. Do not abuse yourself this time around; you are starting with a clean slate.

After returning home, a faster may rarely note some slight swelling around the ankles. This edema resolves rapidly. Fatigue may also be experienced for a few weeks.

If you feel you are too thin, you might be. It's better not to gain the weight back too quickly because you want to build muscle and not fat. Some people are not too thin after the fast. Now, they are just right. However, their friends and family may judge them to be too thin, usually because they themselves are fatter and a lean body makes them uncomfortable by comparison.

Others may also be uncomfortable with the new healthy you. You are eating differently and some may feel threatened or criticized when they realize you are not indulging with them in the American pastime of digging our graves with our knives and forks.

Now is the time to allow the process of healing started by the fast to continue unchecked. Stay with the healthiest diet possible. I regularly see patients who have benefited from a fast continue to heal and make significant gains in health soon afterwards. They continue their recovery while eating, when they weren't able to do so in the past, because the body works more efficiently once the fast gets the ball rolling in the right direction.

Most patients do so well they aim to convert everyone they know. I advise you not to do this unless asked. Live your own life. Let your friends and family listen to tapes or read some books if they are interested. We can help only those who want to help themselves.

Certainly this method of healing is not for everyone. Many will not want to live a healthy life in the face of so much temptation in the modern world. We must respect one's right to choose a lifestyle. But remember, once you have gained the knowledge, your health and happiness are in your hands.

No matter how much money you have—or fame or riches— no possession is so valuable or taken so much for granted as good health. Happiness cannot be achieved without adequate health. It matters not whether you are a multi-millionaire or are unemployed and homeless. You can still find yourself in an intensive care unit or an emergency room of a hospital with tubes in multiple orifices after a medical tragedy. Too often these tragedies occur because of our own doing. If this book convinces you of anything, the most valuable message is: You must earn your good health, it cannot be bought.

I wish you long life and enduring health. It can be yours.

Chapter Notes

Chapter 1

1. Fukudo S, Suzuki J, Nomura T, Iwahashi S, Muranaka M, Taguchi F. Effects of fasting therapy on liver function disorders. *Japanese Journal of Psychosomatic Medicine* 1988;28(6):515–523.
2. Chiba T. Fasting therapy for psychosomatic disorders. *Kango Gijutsu* (Japan) 1985;31(9):1248–9.
3. Bock D, Kohle K, Weimann G, Thomas W, Mente F, Schmidt T, Jaeger M. Prospective studies of the relationship between psychological and social symptoms with the long-term success of hospital fasting therapy. *Verhandlungen Der Deutschen Gesellschaft Fur Innere Medizin* (Germany) 1978;84:1565–7.
4. Yamamoto H. An electro encephalographic study of fasting therapy with special reference to electro encephalographic power spectral changes. *Japanese Journal of Psychosomatic Medicine* 1980;20(4):325–335.
5. Yamamoto H, Suzuki J, Yamauchi Y. Psycho-physiological study on fasting therapy. Symposium on Strategies in Psychosomatic Practice and Research at the 12th European Conference on Psychosomatic Research, Bodo, Norway, July 1987. *Psychotherapy and Psychosomatics* 1979;32(1–4):229–240.
6. Yashiro N. Clinico-psychological and pathophysiological studies on fasting therapy. *Sapporo Medical Journal* (Japan) 1986;55(2):125–136.
7. Suzuki J, Yamauchi Y, Yamamoto H, Komuro U. Fasting therapy for psychosomatic disorders in Japan. *Psychotherapy and Psychosomatics* (Switzerland) 1979;31(1–4):307–314.
8. Suzuki M, Kamijo K. The hypothalamic pituitary adrenal function in mal-nutrition: A comparison between psycho-somatic diseases treated

with fasting therapy and anorexia nervosa. *Folia Endocrinolica Japan* 1979;55(6):739–760.

Chapter 2

1. Berkel J, de Waard F. Mortality pattern and life expectancy of Seventh-Day Adventists in the Netherlands. *International Journal of Epidemiology* 1983;12:455–459.

2. Snowdon DA. Animal product consumption and mortality because of all causes combined, coronary heart disease, stroke, diabetes, and cancer in Seventh-Day Adventists. *American Journal of Clinical Nutrition* 1988;48:739–48.

3. Campbell TC. A study on diet, nutrition and disease in the People's Republic of China. Division of Nutritional Sciences, Cornell University, Ithaca, New York, 1989; pp. 1–9.

4. Saxton JA. Nutrition and growth and their influence on longevity in rats. *Biological Symposium* 1943;11:177.

5. Staszewski J. Age at menarche and breast cancer. *Journal of the National Cancer Institute* 1971;47:935.

6. Masoro EJ, Shimokawa I, Yu BP. Retardation of the aging process in rats by food restriction. *Annals of the New York Academy of Science* 1990;337–52.

7. Goodrick CL, Ingram DK, Reynolds MA, Freeman JR, Cider NL. Effects of intermittent feeding upon growth, activity and lifespan in rats allowed voluntary exercise. *Experimental Aging Research* 1983;9:1477–94.

8. Marston R. Nutrient content of the national food supply. *National Food Review*, U.S.D.A. Dec. 1978, pp. 28–33.

9. Berenson GS, et al. Atherosclerosis of the aorta and coronary arteries and cardiovascular risk factors in persons aged 6 to 30 years and studied at necropsy (The Bogalusa Heart Study). *American Journal of Cardiology* 1992;70:851–858.

10. Carroll KK. Experimental evidence of dietary factors and hormone-dependent cancers. *Cancer Research* 1975;37:3374–83.

11. Berg J. Can nutrition explain the pattern of international epidemiology of hormone-dependent cancer? *Cancer Research* 1975;35:3345.

12. Barone J, Hebert JR, Reddy MM. Dietary fat and natural-killer-cell activity. *American Journal of Clinical Nutrition* 1989;50:861–67.

13. Kozlovsky AS, et al. Effects of diets high in simple sugars on urinary chromium losses. *Metabolism* 1986;35:515.

14. Williams RD, Mason HL, Powers MH, Wilder RM. Induced thiamine deficiency in man: Relation of depletion of thiamine to de-

velopment of biochemical defect and of polyneuropathy. *Archives of Internal Medicine* 1943;71:38–53.

15. Lonsdale D, Shamberger RJ. Red cell transketolase as an indicator of nutritional deficiency. *American Journal of Clinical Nutrition* 1980;33:205–211.

16. Lane BC. Myopia prevention and reversal: New data confirms the interaction of accommodative stress and deficit inducing nutrition. *Journal of the International Academy of Preventative Medicine* 1982;7(3):28.

17. Chen J, Campbell TC, Li J, Peto R. *A Study of Diet Nutrition and Disease in the People's Republic of China.* University of Oxford Press, Cornell University Press, China Publishing House, 1988.

18. Bernard N. An interview with Colin Campbell, MS., Ph. D. April 22, 1994. *Good Medicine* 1994;3:11–14.

19. Diet, nutrition and cancer: Executive summary. *Cancer Research* 1983;43:3020.

20. Lane BC. Myopia prevention and reversal.

21. Herter CA, Kendall AI. The influence of dietary alteration on the types of intestinal flora. *Journal of Biochemical Chemistry* 1909–10;7:216.

22. Korenchevsky V. Autointoxication and processes of aging. *Texas Reports in Biology and Medicine* 1956;12:1016.

23. Horning EC, Dalgliesle CE. The association of skatole forming bacteria in the small intestine with malabsorption syndrome and certain anemias. *Biochemical Journal* 1958;7:13.

24. Select Committee on Nutrition and Human Needs, U.S. Senate. *Dietary Goals for the U.S.* U.S. Government Printing Office, Washington D.C., 1977.

25. Lands WEM, Hamazaki T, Yamakazi K, Okuyama H, Sakai K, Goto Y, Hubbard VS. Changing dietary patterns. *American Journal of Clinical Nutrition* 1990;51:991–3.

26. Wynder EL, Fujita Y, Harris RE, Hirayama T, Hiyama T. Comparative epidemiology of cancer between the United States and Japan. *Cancer* 1991;67:746–63.

27. Phillips RI, Garfinkel L, Kuzma JW, Beeson WL, Lotz TL, Brin B. Mortality among California Seventh-Day Adventists for selected cancer sites. *Journal of the National Cancer Institute* 1980;65:1097–1107.

28. Dunphy J. Etiologic factors in polyposis and carcinoma of the colon. *Annals of Surgery* 1959;150:488.

29. Armstrong B. Environmental factors and cancer incidence and mortality in different countries, with special reference to dietary practices. *International Journal of Cancer* 1975;15:617.

30. Kirshner M. The role of hormones in the etiology of human breast cancer. *Cancer* 1977;39:2716.

31. Ingram DM, Bennett FC, Willcox D, de Clerk N. Effect of low-fat diet on female sex hormone levels. *Journal of the National Cancer Institute* 1987;79(6):1225–9.

32. Staszewski J. Age at menarche and breast cancer. *Journal of the National Cancer Institute* 1971;47:935.

33. Tanner JM. Trend towards earlier menarche in London, Oslo, Copenhagen, the Netherlands and Hungary. *Nature* 1973;243:75–6.

34. Beaton G. *Practical Population Indicators of Health and Nutrition.* World Health Organization monograph, 1976;62:500.

35. Kagawa Y. Impact of westernization on the nutrition of Japanese: Changes in physique, cancer, longevity and centenarians. *Preventative Medicine* 1978;7:205–17.

36. U.S. Department of Health and Human Services. *Surgeon General's Report on Nutrition and Health.* Department of Health and Human Services Publication No. 88–50210, 1988.

37. Mayne ST. Dietary beta carotene and lung cancer risk in U.S. nonsmokers. *Journal of the National Cancer Institute* 1994;86:33.

38. Block F. Epidemiologic evidence regarding vitamin C and cancer. *American Journal of Clinical Nutrition* 1991;54:1310S–1314S.

39. Phillips RL. Role of life-style and dietary habits in risk of cancer among Seventh-Day Adventists. *Cancer Research* 1975;35:3513–3522.

40. Willet WC, Hunter DJ, Stampfer MJ, et al. Dietary fat and fiber in relation to risk of breast cancer: An 8-year follow-up. *Journal of the American Medical Association* 1992;268:2037–44.

41. Rao PN, Prendiville V, Buxton A, Moss DG, Blacklock NJ. Dietary management of urinary risk factor in renal stone formers. *British Journal of Urology* 1982;54:578–83.

42. Hegsted M, Linkswiler HM. Long-term effects of level of protein intake on calcium metabolism in young adult women. *Journal of Nutrition* 1981;111:244–51.

43. Robertson WG, Heyburn PJ, Peacock M, Hanes FA, Swaminathan R. The effect of high animal protein intake on the risk of calcium stone formation in the urinary tract. *Clinical Science* 1979:57:285–88.

44. Zemel MB, Schuette SA, Hegsted M, Linkswiler HM. Role of sulfur-containing amino acids in protein induced hypercalciuria in men. *Journal of Nutrition* 1981;111:545–52.

45. Mazess RB, Mather W. Bone mineral content of North American Eskimos. *American Journal of Clinical Nutrition* 1974;27:916–925.

46. O'Connell JM, Dibley MJ, Sierra J, Wallace B, Marks JS, Yip R. Growth of vegetarian children: The farm study. *Pediatrics* 1989;84:475–481.

47. McDougall JA, McDougall MA. *The McDougall Plan.* Piscataway, N.J.: New Century Publishers, 1983, pp. 95–109.

48. Nasset ES. Role of the digestive tract in the utilization of protein and amino acids. *Journal of the American Medical Association* 1957;164(2):172.

49. Allen LH, Oddoye EA, Margen S. Protein-induced hypercalciuria. *American Journal of Clinical Nutrition* 1979;32:741–749.

50. Robertson WG, Peacock M, Hodgkinson A. Dietary changes and the incidence of urinary calculi in the U.K. between 1958 and 1976. *Journal of Chronic Disease* 1979;22:469–476.

51. Corliss J. Pesticide metabolites linked to breast cancer. *Journal of the National Cancer Institute* 1993;85:602.

52. Osborne MP, Bradlow HL, Wong GYC, Telang NT. Up-regulation of estradiol C16-hydroxylation in human breast tissue: A potential biomarker of breast cancer risk. *Journal of the National Cancer Institute* 1993;85:1917–1920.

53. Dietary carcinogens linked to breast cancer. *Medical World News,* May 1993; p.13.

54. Ornish D, et al. Can lifestyle changes reverse coronary heart disease? *Lancet* 1990;336(8708):129–133.

55. United States Department of Agriculture, Economic Research Service. *Provisions of the Food, Agriculture, Conservation, and Trade Act of 1990.* Agriculture Information Bulletin No. 624. Washington, 1991, p. vii.

56. Stare F. *Adventures in Nutrition.* Hanover, Mass.: Christopher Publishing House. 1991, p. 126.

Chapter 3

1. Jennings I. *The Philosophy of Human Life.* Cleveland, 1852; republished in 1960 by Health Research, Mokelumne Hill, California.

2. Tilden JH. *Toxemia, the Basic Cause of Disease.* Tampa, Florida: Natural Hygiene Press, 1974, p. 7-8.

3. Harmon D. Aging: A theory based on free radical and radiation chemistry. *Journal of Gerontology* 1956;11:298–300.

4. Yu BP, Langeniere S, Kim JW. Influence of life-prolonging food restriction on membrane lipoperoxidation and antioxidant status, in *Oxygen Radicals in Biology and Medicine.* Simic, Taylor, Ward, Von Sonntag (eds.): New York: Plenum Pub, 1988, pp. 1067–1073.

5. Bjorksten J. Crosslinkage theory of aging. *Journal of the American Geriatrics Society* 1968;16:408.

6. Holeckova E, Chuapil M. The effects of intermittent feeding and fasting and of domestication on biological age in the rat. *Gerontologia* 1965;11:96.

7. Barrows CH. Nutrition and aging: The time has come to move from laboratory research to clinical studies. *Geriatrics* 1977;32:39.

8. Kent S. Can dietary manipulations prolong life? *Geriatrics* 1978;32:102.

9. Ross MH. Dietary behavior and longevity. *Nutritional Review* 1977;35:257.

10. McCay CM. Effects of retarded feeding upon aging and chronic disease in rats and dogs. *American Journal of Public Health* 1947;37:521.

11. Lindsted K, Tonstad S, Kuzma JW. Body mass index and patterns of mortality among Seventh-Day Adventist men. *International Journal of Obesity* 1991;15:397–406.

12. Simopoulos AP, Van Itallie TB. Body weight: Health and longevity. *Annals of Internal Medicine* 1984;100:285–295.

13. Murray J, Murray A. Suppression of infection by famine and its activation by refeeding—a paradox. *Perspectives in Biology and Medicine* 1977;20:471.

14. McCay CM, Crowell MF, Maynard LA. The effect of retarded growth upon the length of lifespan and upon the ultimate body size. *Journal of Nutrition* 1935;10:63–79.

15. Sprunt DH. The effect of undernourishment on the susceptibility of the rabbit to infection with vaccinia. *Journal of Experimental Medicine* 1942;75:297–304.

16. Gotch FM, Spry CJF, Mowat AG, Beeson PB, Maclennan ICM. Reversible granulocyte killing defect in anorexia nervosa. *Clinical Experiments in Immunology* 1975;21:244–9.

17. Reiger W, Brady JP, Weisberg E. Hematologic changes in anorexia nervosa. *American Journal of Psychology* 1978;135:984–5.

18. Bowers TK, Eckert E. Leukopenia in anorexia nervosa: Lack of increased risk of infection. *Archives of Internal Medicine* 1978; 138:1520–3.

19. Pertschuk MJ, Crosby LO, Barot L, Mullen JL. Immunocompetence in anorexia nervosa. *American Journal of Clinical Nutrition* 1982;35:968–72.

20. Keys A, Brozek J, Henschel A, Mickelson O, Taylor HL. *The Biology of Human Starvation*. Minneapolis: University of Minnesota, 1950.

21. Wing EJ, Stanko RT, Winkelstein A, Abidi SA. Fasting enhanced immune effector mechanism in obese subjects *American Journal of Medicine* 1983;75:91–96.

22. Ruckner C, Hoffman J. *The Seventh-Day Adventist Diet*. New York: Random House, 1991.

23. Snowdon DA. Animal product consumption and mortality because of all causes combined, coronary heart disease, stroke, diabetes,

and cancer in Seventh-Day Adventists. *American Journal of Clinical Nutrition* 1988;48:739–48.

24. Rotkin ID. Studies in the epidemiology of prostate cancer: Expanded sampling. *Cancer Treatment Reports* 1977;61:173–80.

25. Kahn HA, Phillips RL, Snowdon DA, Choi W. Association between reported diet and all causes of mortality: twenty-one-year followup on 27,530 adult Seventh-Day Adventists. *American Journal of Epidemiology* 1984;119:775–87.

Chapter 4

1. Stewart WF, Lipton RB, Celentano DD, Reed ML. Prevalence of migraine headache in the United States. *Journal of the American Medical Association* 1992;267:64–69.

2. Silberstein SD, Silberstein MM. New concepts in the pathogenesis of headache. *Pain Management* September/October 1990, pp. 297–303; November/December 1990, pp. 334–342.

3. Basbaum AI, Levine JD. The contribution of the nervous system to inflammation and inflammatory disease. *Canadian Journal of Physiology and Pharmacology* 1991;69:647–651.

4. Fanciullacci M, Franchi G, Sicuteri F. Hypersensitivity to lysergic acid diethylamide (LSD-25) and psilocybin in essential headache. *Experientia* 1974;30:(1)441.

5. Stephenson J. Detox is crucial in chronic daily headache. *Family Practice News,* July 1, 1993, p. 2.

6. Rapoport AM, Weeks RE, Sheftell FD, Baskin MB, Cob C, Verdi J. The "analgesic washout period": A critical variable in the evaluation of headache treatment efficacy. *Neurology* 1986;36(suppl.):100–101. Abstract.

7. Strategies for migraine prevention, relief. *Family Practice News,* August 15, 1992, p. 1.

8. Merritt JE, Williams PB. Vasospasm contributes to monosodium glutamate-induced headache. *Headache,* September 1990, pp. 575–580.

9. Scopp AL. MSG and hydrolyzed protein induced headaches: Review and case studies. *Headache* 1991;31:107–110.

10. Kerr GR, Wu-Lee M, El-Lozy M, McGandy R, Stare FJ. Prevalence of the "Chinese restaurant syndrome." *Journal of the American Dietetic Association* 1979;75:29–33.

11.Reif-Lehrer L. A questionnaire study of the prevalence of the Chinese restaurant syndrome. *Federation Proceedings* 1977;36:1617–1623.

12.Blank C. The MSG controversy. *Informed Consent* 1994;1:(3) 4–7.

Chapter 5

1. Roberts J, Maurer K. Blood pressure levels of persons 6–74 years, United States, 1971–1974. Department of Health, Education, and Welfare. Publication No. (HRA) 78-1648, Series 11, No. 203 Sept. 1977.

2. Freis E. Salt, volume and the prevention of hypertension. *Circulation* 1976;53:589.

3. Sever P, Peart WS, Gorden D, Beighton P. Blood pressure and its correlates in urban and tribal Africa. *Lancet* 1980;2:60.

4. Connor WE, Connor BL. The key role of nutritional factors in the prevention of coronary heart disease. *Preventative Medicine* 1972;1:49.

5. Stamler J. Lifestyles, major risk factors, proof and public policy. *Circulation* 1978;58:3.

6. Lovastatin for hypercholesterolemia. *The Medical Letter* 1987;29:99–101.

7. Frick HM, Elo O, Haapa K, et al. Helsinki Heart Trial study: Primary-prevention trial with gemfibrozil in middle aged men with dyslipidemia. *New England Journal of Medicine* 1987;317:1237–1245.

8. Luchi RJ, Scott SM, Deupree RH, et al. Comparison of medical and surgical treatment for unstable angina pectoris. *New England Journal of Medicine* 1987; 316:977–984.

9. Winslow CM, Kosecoff JB, Chassin M, et al. The appropriateness of performing coronary artery bypass surgery. *Journal of the American Medical Association* 1988;260:505–509.

10. *Assessing the Efficacy and Safety of Medical Technologies.* Washington DC, Congress of the United States, Office of Technology Assessment Publication No. 052-003-00593-0. Government Printing Office, Washington DC, 1978.

11. Hannan EL, Bernard HR, Kilburn HC, O'Donnell JF. Gender differences in mortality rates for coronary artery bypass surgery. *American Heart Journal* 1992;123:866–872.

12. Editorial: Brain damage and open-heart surgery. *Lancet* Aug. 12, 1989; 364–366.

13. Taylor K. Brian damage during open-heart surgery. *Thorax* 1982;37:873.

14. Orr W. Sleep disturbances after open heart surgery. *American Journal of Cardiology* 1977;39:196.

15. Henriksen L. Evidence suggestive of diffuse brain damage following cardiac operations. *Lancet* 1984;1:816.

16. Cashin LW, Sanmarco ME, Nessim AS, Blankenhorn DH. Accelerated progression of atherosclerosis in coronary vessels with minimal lesions that are bypassed. *New England Journal of Medicine* 1984;311(13):824–828.

17. Meier B, King SB, Gruentzig AR, et al. Repeat coronary angioplasty. *Journal of the American College of Cardiology* 1984;4:463.

18. Ornish D, Brown SE, Scherwitz LW, et al. Can lifestyle changes reverse coronary heart disease? *Lancet* 1990;336(8708):129–133.

19. Kahn JK. Reversing coronary atherosclerosis. *Postgraduate Medicine* 1993;94(1):50–65.

20. Carpi J. Low-fat diet can keep arteries young and disease-free. *Medical Tribune,* November 25, 1993, p. 3.

21. Ellis F. Angina and vegan diet. *American Heart Journal* 1977;1:93(6):803–4.

22. Blankenhorn DH, Nessim SA, Johnson RL, et al. Beneficial effects of combined colestipol-niacin therapy on coronary atherosclerosis and coronary venous bypass grafts. *Journal of the American Medical Association* 1987;257:3233.

23. Wenxun F, Parker R, Parpia B, et al. Erythrocyte fatty acids, plasma lipids and cardiovascular disease in rural China. *American Journal of Clinical Nutrition* 1990;52:1027–32.

24. Brody J. Huge study of diet indicts fat and meat. *New York Times,* May 8, 1990, "Science Times" section, p. 1.

25. Diet and disease: The China Study. *Health Science,* September/October 1992, p. 8.

26. West K. *Epidemiology of Diabetes and Its Vascular Lesions.* New York: Elsevier, 1978, p. 353–402.

27. Freis E. Salt, volume and the prevention of hypertension. *Circulation* 1976;53:589.

28. Himsworth H. Diet in the aetiology of human diabetes. *Proceedings of the Royal Society of Medicine* 1949;42:323.

29. Ramsey LE, Yeo WW, Jackson PR. Dietary reduction of serum cholesterol concentration: Time to think again. *British Medical Journal* 1991;303:953–957.

30. O'Brien BC, Reiser R. Human plasma lipid responses to red meat, poultry, fish, and eggs. *American Journal of Clinical Nutrition* 1980;33:2573–2580.

31. Flynn MA, Naumann HD, Nolph GB, Krause G, Ellersieck M. Dietary "meats" and serum lipids. *American Journal of Clinical Nutrition* 1982;35:935–942.

32. McDougall JA. Is the cholesterol scare a scam? *Vegetarian Times,* December 1989, pp. 56–69.

33. Sacks F. Ingestion of egg raises plasma-low-density lipoproteins in free-living subjects. *Lancet* 1984;1:647–649.

34. McMurry M. The absorption of cholesterol and the sterol balance in the Tarahumara Indians of Mexico fed cholesterol-free and high-

cholesterol diets. *American Journal of Clinical Nutrition* 1985;41:1289–1298.

35. Sorbris R, Aly KO, Nilsson-Ehle P, Petersson BG, Ockerman PA. Vegetarian fasting of obese patients: A clinical and biochemical evaluation. *Scandinavian Journal of Gastroenterology* 1982;17:417–24.

36. Vessby B, Boberg M, Karlstrom B, Lithell H, Werner I. et al. Improved metabolic control after supplemented fasting in overweight type 2 diabetic patients. *Acta Medica Scandinavica* 1984;216:67–274.

37. Brozek J, Wells S, Keys A. Medical aspect of semi-starvation in Leningrad. *American Review of Soviet Medicine* 1946–7;4:70–86.

38. Wanscher O, Clemmesen J, Nielsen A. Negative correlation between atherosclerosis and carcinoma. *British Journal of Cancer* 1951;5:1345–1354.

39. Gresham GA. Is atheroma a reversible lesion? *Atherosclerosis* 1976;23:379–391.

40. Armstrong ML. Evidence of regression of atherosclerosis in primates and man. *Postgraduate Medical Journal* 1976;52:456–461.

41. Hopf R. Gleubner M, Babej-Dolle R, Kaltenbach M. Wirksamkeit von chelat bei patienten mit koronarer herzkrankheit. *German Journal of Cardiology* 1987;79(suppl. 2):73.

42. Diehm C. "Wundermittel Chelat" anspruch und wirklichkeit. *Zeitschrift der Deutschen Herzstiftung* 1986;10:11–15.

43. Sloth-Nielsen J, Guldager B, Mouritzen C, Lund EB, Egeblad M, Norregaard O, Jorgensen SJ, Jelnes R. Arteriographic findings in EDTA chelation therapy on peripheral arteriosclerosis. *American Journal of Surgery* 1991;162:122–125.

44. Guldager B, Jelnes R, Jorgenson SJ, Nielsen JS, Klerke A, Mogensen K, Larsens KE, Reimer E, Holm J, Ottesen S. EDTA treatment of intermittent claudication—a double blind, placebo-controlled study. *Journal of Internal Medicine* 1992;231:261–267.

45. Duncan GG, Cristofori FC, Yue JK, Murthy MSJ. The control of obesity by intermittent fasts. *Medical Clinics of North America* 1964;48:1359–1372.

46. Suzuki J, Yamauchi Y, Horikawa M, Yamagata S. Fasting therapy for psychosomatic diseases with special reference to its indication and therapeutic mechanism. *Tohoku Journal of Experimental Medicine* (suppl) 1976;118:245–259.

47. Krotkiewski M, Ruzyllo E, Kotowska A. Obesity and arterial hypertension: II. Effect of a reducing diet and fasting. *Polish Medical Science and History* 1967;10:58–62.

48. Goldhamer A. The effect of water fasting on hypertension (study in progress). Center for Conservative Therapy, Pengrove, Cal. Personal communication, August 30, 1994.

49. Bloom WL, Azar G, Smith EG. Changes in heart size and plasma volume during fasting. *Metabolism.* 1966;15:409–413.

50. Haxhe JJ. Experimental undernutrition: I. Its effects on cardiac output. *Metabolism* 1967;16:1086–91.

51. Rouse IL, Beilin LJ, Armstrong BK, Vandongen R. Blood pressure lowering effects of vegetarian diet: Controlled trial in normotensive subjects. *Lancet* 1983;1:5–9.

52. Douglass J, Rasgon IM, Fleiss PM, et al. Effects of a raw food diet on hypertension and obesity. *Southern Medical Journal* 1985;78(7):841.

53. Kannel WB. *Coronary Risk Handbook: Estimating Risk of Coronary Heart Disease in Daily Practice.* New York: American Heart Association, 1973.

54. Ames RP. Antihypertensive therapy and risk factors for coronary heart disease. *Practical Cardiology* 1989;15:49–66.

55. Yusuf S, Wittes J, Friedman L. Overview of results of randomized clinical trials in heart disease. *Journal of the American Medical Association* 1988;260:2259–2263.

56. Muliar LA, Mishchenko VP, Loban GA, Goncharenko LL, Bobyrev VN. Effect of complete fasting on the coagulative and antioxidative properties of blood. *Voprosy Pitaniya* July-August 1984;4:20–23. (ISSN 0042-8833. Journal Code: XK4. Language: Russian. Summary language: English.)

57. Miettinen M. Effect of fasting on fibrinolysis and blood coagulation. *American Journal of Cardiology* 1962;10:532–534.

58. Menon IS. Fasting and non-fasting fibrinolytic activity. *Laboratory Practice* 1967;16:469–470.

59. Lawlor T, Wells DG. Metabolic hazards of fasting. *American Journal of Clinical Nutrition* 1969;22:1142–1148.

60. Stechschulte D. Dunn M. Starvation and heart failure. *Journal of the Kansas Medical Society,* November 1965, pp. 500–502.

61. Merrill AJ. Intractable heart failure management with 5–7 days of fasting, a preliminary trial. *American Heart Journal* 1964;67:433–436.

62. Bloom WL, Mitchell W. Salt excretion of fasting patients. *Archives of Internal Medicine* 1960; 106:321–326.

63. Weinsier RL. Fasting: A review with emphasis on the electrolytes. *American Journal of Medicine* 1971;50:233–240.

Chapter 6

1. Howard BV. Lipoprotein metabolism in diabetes mellitus. *Journal of Lipid Research* 1987;28:613–628.

2. Insulin therapy may promote atherosclerosis. *Family Practice News,* March 1, 1992, p. 42.

3. Kahn JK. Reversing coronary atherosclerosis. *Postgraduate Medicine* 1993;94:50–65.

4. Carre J. Low-fat diet can keep arteries young and disease-free. *Medicine Tribune,* November 25, 1993, p. 3.

5. Wenxun F, Parker R, Parpia B, et al. Erythrocyte fatty acids, plasma lipids and cardiovascular disease in rural China. *American Journal of Clinical Nutrition* 1990;52:1027–32.

6. West K. *Epidemiology of Diabetes and Its Vascular Lesions.* New York: Elsevier, 1978, pp. 353–402.

7. Sweeney J. Dietary factors that influence the dextrose tolerance test: A preliminary study. *Archives of Internal Medicine* 1927;40:818.

8. Hollenbeck C, Donner CC, Williams RA, Reaven GM. The effects of variations in percent of naturally occurring complex and simple carbohydrates on plasma glucose and insulin response in individuals with non-insulin dependent diabetes mellitus. *Diabetes* 1985;34:151.

9. To preserve their health and heritage, Arizona Indians reclaim ancient foods. *New York Times,* May 21, 1991, pp. C1,C10.

10. Himsworth H. Diet in the etiology of human diabetes. *Proceedings of the Royal Society of Medicine* 1949;42:323–326.

11. Kawate R. Diabetes mellitus and its vascular complications in Japanese migrants on the island of Hawaii. *Diabetes Care* 1979;2:161–170.

12. Insulin therapy may promote atherosclerosis. *Family Practice News.*

13. Zoler LZ. Insulin therapy discouraged in type II diabetes patients. *Family Practice News,* Sept. 15, 1993, pp. 1,26.

14. Berger W. Incidence of severe side effects during therapy with sulfonylureas and biguanides. *Hormone and Metabolic Research Supplement* 1985;15:111–5.

15. Boyd AE. Sulfonylurea receptors, ion channels, and fruit flies. *Diabetes* 1988;37:847–50.

16. Kolterman OG, Gray RS, Shapiro G, et al. The acute and chronic effects of sulfonylurea therapy in type II diabetic subjects. *Diabetes* 1984;33:346–54.

17. Snowdon DA. Animal product consumption and mortality because of all causes combined, coronary heart disease, stroke, diabetes, and cancer in Seventh-Day Adventists. *American Journal of Clinical Nutrition* 1988;48:739–48.

18. Kahn HA, Phillips RL, Snowdon DA, Chop W. Association between reported diet and all-cause mortality. *American Journal of Epidemiology* 1984;119(5):775–787.

19. Paolisso GP, D'Amore A, Giugliano D, et al. Pharmacologic doses

of vitamin E improve insulin action in healthy subjects and non-insulin dependent diabetic patients. *American Journal of Clinical Nutrition* 1993;57:650–656.

20. Davie S, Gould B, Yudkin J. Effect of vitamin C on glycosylation of proteins. *Diabetes* 1992;41:167–173.

21. Allen FM. Prolonged fasting in diabetes. *American Journal of the Medical Sciences* 1915;159(4):480–485.

22. Vessby B, Boberg M, Karlstrom B, et al. Improved metabolic control after supplemented fasting in overweight type II diabetic patients *Acta Medica Scandinavia* 1984;216:67–74.

23. McCarty MF. Maturity-onset diabetes—toward a physiologically appropriate management. *Medical Hypothesis* (England) 1981;7(10): 1265–1285.

24. Gueris J, Segrestaa JM, Lamotte M. Insulinemia in the obese before and after fasting therapy. *Journal Annuel Diabetologie Hotel Dieu* (France) 1969;10:287–292.

Chapter 7

1. Halla JR, Volanakis JE, Schrohenloher RE. Immune complexes in rheumatoid arthritis sera and synovial fluids. *Arthritis and Rheumatism* 1979;22(5):440–448.

2. Paganelli R, Levinsky RJ, Brostoff J, Wraith DG. Immune complexes containing food proteins in normal and atopic subjects after oral challenges and effect of sodium chromoglycate on antigen absorption. *Lancet* 1979;1:1270–1272.

3. Panush RS. Delayed reactions to foods: Food allergy and rheumatic disease. *Annals of Allergy* 1986;56:500–503.

4. Palmblad J. Lymphomas and dietary fat. *Lancet* 1977;1:142.

5. *Physician's Compendium of Drug Therapy.* Secaucus, N.J.: Compendium Publications Group, 1993, 8:2–8.

6. Bjarnason I, Williams P, So A, et al. Intestinal permeability and inflammation in rheumatoid arthritis: Effects of nonsteroidal anti-inflammatory drugs. *Lancet* Nov 24, 1984;1171–1174.

7. *Goodman and Gilman's The Pharmacologic Basis of Therapeutics,* ed. 6. New York: Macmillan, 1980, pp. 1482–1487.

8. *Physician's Compendium of Drug Therapy,* 1993;8:18.

9. *Goodman and Gilman's The Pharmacologic Basis of Therapeutics,* ed. 6. New York: Macmillan, 1980, p. 1276.

10. *Physician's Compendium of Drug Therapy,* 1993;8:40.

11. Blocka K, Paulus HE. The clinical pharmacology of the gold compounds, in Paulus, et al. (eds.): *Drugs for Rheumatic Diseases.* New York: Longman (Churchill Livingstone), 1987, pp. 49–83.

12. *Goodman and Gilman's The Pharmacologic Basis of Therapeutics,* 1980, p. 1046.

13. Beck M, Hager M, Smith VE. Living with arthritis. *Newsweek,* March 20, 1989, pp. 64, 70.

14. Pincus T. New concepts in prognosis of rheumatic disease for the 1990's, in Bellamy N (ed.): *Prognosis in the Rheumatic Diseases.* Boston: Kluwer Academic, 1991, pp. 451–92.

15. Brooks PM, Buchanan WW. Prediction of the clinical efficacy of and intolerance to antirheumatic drug therapy, in Bellamy N (ed.): *Prognosis in the Rheumatic Disease.* Boston: Kluwer Academic, 1991, pp. 347–402.

16. Kushner I. Does aggressive therapy of rheumatoid arthritis affect outcome? *The Journal of Rheumatology* 1989;16:1–4.

17. Scott D, Coulton BL, Symmons DMP, Popert AJ. Long-term outcome of treating rheumatoid arthritis: Results after 20 years. *Lancet* May 16, 1987;1108–1111.

18. Beighton P, Solomon L, Valkenburg HA, et al. Rheumatoid arthritis in a rural South African Negro population. *Annals of Rheumatologic Diseases* 1975;34:136.

19. Beasley R, Bennett PH, Lin CC. Low prevalence of rheumatoid arthritis in Chinese: Prevalence survey in a rural community. *Journal of Rheumatology* 1983;10(Suppl 10):11.

20. Morrow WJW, Levy JA. Dietary fat and autoimmune disease. *Arthritis and Rheumatism* 1983;26:1532.

21. Solomon L. Rheumatic disorders in South African Negro: Part I. Rheumatoid arthritis and ankylosing spondylitis. *South African Medical Journal* 1975;49:1292.

22. Lucas P, Power L. Dietary fat aggravates active rheumatoid arthritis. *Clinical Research* 1981;29:754A.

23. Uden A, Trang L, Venizelos N, Palmblad J. Neutrophil functions and clinical performance after total fasting in patients with rheumatoid arthritis. *Annals of Rheumatological Diseases* 1983;42:45–51.

24. Skoldstam L, Larsson L, Lindstorm FD. Effects of fasting and lactovegetarian diet on rheumatoid arthritis. *Scandinavian Journal of Rheumatology* 1979;8:249–255.

25. Kroker GF, Stroud RM, Marshall R, et al. Fasting and rheumatoid arthritis: A multicenter study. *Clinical Ecology* 1984;2(3):137–144.

26. Hafstrom I, Ringertz B, Gyllenhammar H, Palmblad J, Harms-Ringdahl M. Effects of fasting on disease activity, neutrophil function, fatty acid composition, and leukotriene biosynthesis in patients with rheumatoid arthritis. *Arthritis and Rheumatism* 1988;31:585.

27. Kjeldsen-Kragh J, Haugen M, Borchgrevink CF, et al. Controlled

trial of fasting and one year vegetarian diet in rheumatoid arthritis. *Lancet* 1991;338:899–902.

28. Panush RS, Stroud RM, Webster EM. Food-induced allergic arthritis. *Arthritis and Rheumatism* 1986;29(2):220–226.

29. Faivelson S. Vegetable diet may improve autoimmune disease. *Medical Tribune,* June 11, 1992, p. 32.

30. Faivelson S. Generalists can offer patients state-of-the-art treatment options for rheumatoid arthritis. *Medical Tribune,* Oct. 23, 1992, p. 2

31. Faivelson S, p. 32.

32. Hafstrom I, et al.

33. Lithell H, Bruce A, Gustafsson IB, et al. A fasting and vegetarian diet treatment trial on chronic inflammatory disorders: Effects on clinical condition and serum levels of neutrophil-derived granule proteins. *Acta Dermato-Venereologia* (Stockholm) 1983;63:397.

34. Wofy D. New approaches treating systematic lupus erythematosus. *Western Journal of Medicine* 1987;147:181–6.

35. Bullard-Dillard R, Chen J, Pelsue S, Dao V, Agris PF. Anti-Sm autoantibodies of systematic lupus erythematosus cross react with dietary plant proteins. *Immunological Investigations* 1992;21(3):193–202.

36. Roberts J. Exacerbation of SLE associated with alfalfa ingestion. *New England Journal of Medicine* 1983;308:1361.

37. Aladjem H. *Understanding Lupus.* New York: Charles Scribner's Sons, 1982, pp. 46–49.

38. Krieg AM. Environmental factors and lupus. *Lupus News* 1992;11(3).

39. Hochberg MC. Systemic lupus erythematosus. *Rheumatic Diseases Clinics of North America* 1990;16(3):617–639.

40. Reidenberg MM. Aromatic amines and the pathogenesis of lupus erythematosus. *American Journal of Medicine* 1983;75:1037.

41. Agris PF. North Carolina State University Department of Biochemistry. Personal communication, August 26, 1994.

42. Corman L. The role of diet in animal models of systemic lupus erythematosus: Possible implications for human lupus. *Seminars in Arthritis and Rheumatism* 1985;15(1):61–69.

43. Morrow WJW, Yovinov P, Isenberg DA, Snaith ML. Systemic lupus erythematosus: 25 years of treatment related to immunopathology. *Lancet* 1983;2(8343):206–210.

44. Fessel WJ. Epidemiology of systemic lupus erythematosus. *Rheumatic Diseases Clinics of North America* 1988;14(1):15–23.

45. Aladjem H. *Understanding Lupus,* pp. 40–43.

46. Shigemasa C, Tanaka T, Mashiba H. Effect of vegetarian diet on systemic lupus erythematosus. *Lancet* 1992;339:1177.

47. Schmeck HM. Baffling rise of intestinal disorder in the young. *New York Times,* Dec. 1, 1988, p. B23.

48. Hanson LA, Ahistedt S, Anderson B, et al. Protective factors in milk and the development of the immune system. *Pediatrics* 1985;75(suppl):172–176.

49. Foucard T. Development of food allergies with special reference to cow's milk allergy. *Pediatrics* 1985;75(suppl):177–181.

50. Acheson ED, Truelove SC. Early weaning in the aetiology of ulcerative colitis. *British Medical Journal* 1961;2:929–931.

51. Whorwell PJ, Holdstock G, Whorwell GM, Wright R. Bottle feeding, early gastroenteritis and inflammatory bowel disease. *British Medical Journal* 1979;1:382–383.

52. Truelove SC. Ulcerative colitis provoked by milk. *British Medical Journal* 1961;1:154–160.

53. Faber J, Zaides S, Kuperman O, et al. Lymphocyte response to a bovine milk protein in ulcerative colitis. *Israel Journal of Medical Sciences* 1985;21:575–578.

54. Farmer RG. Infectious causes of diarrhea in the differential diagnosis of inflammatory disease. *Medical Clinics of North America* 1990;74:29–38.

55. Jones A, Workman AE, Freeman AH, Dickinson RJ, Wilson AJ, Hunter JO. Crohn's disease: Maintenance of remission by diet. *Lancet* 1985;2:177–180.

56. VonBrandes JW, Lorenz-Meyer H. Diet excluding refined sugar: A new perspective for the treatment of Crohn's disease? A randomized controlled study. *Zeitschrift für Gastroenterologie* 1981;19:1–12.

57. Afonso JJ, Rombeau JL. Nutritional care for patients with Crohn's disease. *Hepatogastroenterology* 1990;37(1):32–41.

58. Riordan A, Hunter JO, Cowan RE, et al. Treatment of active Crohn's disease by exclusion diet: East Anglian Multicenter Controlled Trial. *Lancet* 1993;342:1131–4.

59. Heaton K, Thorton JR, Emmett, PM. Treatment of Crohn's Disease with an unrefined-carbohydrate, fiber-rich diet. *British Medical Journal* 1979;2:764.

60. Spiller G, Freeman HJ. Recent advances in dietary fiber and colorectal diseases. *American Journal of Clinical Nutrition* 1981;34:1145.

61. Darlington LG, Ramsey NW, Mansfield JR. Placebo-controlled, blind study of dietary manipulation in rheumatoid arthritis. *Lancet* 1986;1:236–238.

62. Stroud RM. The effect of fasting followed by specific food challenges on rheumatoid arthritis, in Hahn BH, Arnett FC, Zizic TM (eds.): *Current Topics in Rheumatology:* Upjohn, 1983, pp. 145–157.

63. Solomon P, Kornbluth AA, Janowitz HD. Treatment of ulcerative

colitis with fish oils in omega fatty acid: An open trial. *Journal of Clinical Gastroenterology* 1990;12:157–161.

64. Greenberg GR, Fleming CR, Jeejeebhoy KN, et al. Controlled trial of bowel rest and nutritional support in the management of Crohn's disease. *Gut* 1988;29(10):1309–15.

Chapter 8

1. Sears MR, Taylor DR, Print CG, et al. Regular inhaled beta-agonist treatment in bronchial asthma. *Lancet* 1990;336:1391–1396.

2. Mullen M, Mullen B, Carey M. The association between B-agonist use and death from asthma. *Journal of the American Medical Association* 1993;279:1842–1845.

3. Dzhugostran VI, Niamtse ET, Zlepka VD, Marchenko IG. Enterosorption and therapeutic fasting in the treatment of patients with bronchial asthma. *Klin Med* (Moscow) 1991;69(4):54–56.

4. Gorbachev VV, Sytyi VP, Sizova EP, Vasnev VI, Boyarintseva AV. Use of controlled therapeutic fasting in bronchial asthma. *Adravookhr Beloruss* 1979;0(9):55–58.

5. Kokosov AN, Osinin SG, Faustova ME. The fasting dietetic therapy as a non-medicamentous method of choice in complicated cases of asthmatic bronchitis and bronchial asthma: Pathophysiological shifts, indications for treatment, results (a review of the reported data including own studies). *Terapevticheski Arkhiv,* Moscow 1991. Recorded at National Library of Medicine, code 1991;63(3):100–103, 107.

6. Braitman L, Aldin EV, Stanton JL. Obesity and caloric intake. The National Health and Nutrition Examination Survey of 1971–1975. *Journal of Chronic Disease* 1985;38:727–732.

7. Kromhout D. Energy and macronutrient intake in lean and obese middle-aged men. *American Journal of Clinical Nutrition* 1983;37:295–299.

8. Niederpreum M, Miller WC, Lindeman AK, Wallace J. Contribution of dietary fat to body fatness in lean and obese adults. *Medical Science of Sports and Exercise* 1990;22:S129.

9. Foryet J, Goodrick GK, Gotto AM. Limitations of behavioral treatment of obesity: Review and analysis. *Journal of Behavioral Medicine* 1981;4:159–173.

10. Liquid protein and sudden death. *FDA Drug Bulletin* 1978:8;18–19.

11. Center for Disease Control. *Liquid Protein Diets.* U.S. Public Health Service. 1979 Publication No. EPI-78-11-2.

12. Shelton HM. *Fasting Can Save Your Life.* Tampa, Fl.: American Natural Hygiene Society, 1993, p. 21.

Chapter 9

1. Salloum TK, Burton A. Therapeutic fasting, in Pizzorno JE, Murray MT (eds.): *A Textbook of Natural Medicine*. Seattle: John Bastyr College Publications: 1987.

2. Owen OE, Morgan AP, Kemp HG, et al. Brain metabolism during fasting. *Journal of Clinical Investigation* 1967;46:1589–1595.

3. Yamamoto H, Suzuki J, Yamauchi Y. Psychophysiological study of fasting therapy. *Psychotherapy and Psychosomatics* (Switzerland) 1979;32(1–4):229–240.

4. Bloom WL. Fasting as an introduction to the treatment of obesity. *Metabolism* 1959;8(May):515–520.

5. Salloum TK. *Fasting Signs and Symptoms: A Clinical Guide*. East Palestine, Ohio: Buckey Naturopathic Press, 1992.

6. Keys A, Brozek J, Henschel A, et al. *The Biology of Human Starvation*, vol. 1 and 2. Minneapolis: University of Minnesota Press, 1950.

7. Shelton HM. *The Science and Fine Art of Fasting*. Chicago: Natural Hygiene Press, 1978.

8. Drenick EJ, Swendseid ME, Blahd WH, Tuttle SG. Prolonged starvation as treatment for severe obesity. *Journal of the American Medical Association* 1964;187:100–105.

9. Lawlor T, Wells DG. Metabolic hazards of fasting. *American Journal of Clinical Nutrition* 1969;22:1142–1148.

10. McCarty DJ. Gout without hyperuricemia. *Journal of the American Medical Association* 1994;271:302.

11. Cahill GF. Famine Symposium: Physiology of acute starvation in man. *Ecology of Food and Nutrition* 1978;6:221–230.

12. Barrett PVD. Hyperbilirubinemia of fasting. *Journal of the American Medical Association* 1971;271(10): 1349–1353.

13. Sorbris R, Aly KO, Nilsson-Ehle BG, Peterson G, Ockerman PA. Vegetarian fasting of obese patients: A clinical and biochemical evaluation. *Scandinavian Journal of Gastroenterology* 1982;17:417–424.

14. Garnett ES, Barnard DL, Ford J, et al. Gross fragmentation of cardiac myofibrils after therapeutic starvation for obesity. *Lancet* 1969;1:914–916.

15. Kahan A. Death during therapeutic starvation. *Lancet* 1968;1:1378–1379.

16. Spencer IOB. Death during therapeutic starvation for obesity. *Lancet* 1968;1:1288–1290.

Index

anti-inflammatory substances, natural, 171
antioxidants, 26, 29, 37, 64–65, 110, 129, 138
anxiety, 19, 28, 89, 93, 151
apoproteins, 37
appendicitis, 30, 112
appetite, loss of, 8, 14, 68
apples, 55, 167
arsenic, 80
arthrectomy, 102, 105, 119
arthritis, 1, 20, 157, 171. *See also* rheumatoid arthritis
aspirin, 150, 201
asthma, 20, 144, 178–82; case history, 180–82
atherosclerosis, 22, 24, 101–2, 104–5, 127, 128, 130; case history, 113–15. *See also* plaque, atherosclerotic
atherosclerotic lesions, 28–29
atrial fibrillation, 203–4
autoantibody production, 161–62
autoimmune diseases, 9, 39, 52, 63, 143–72, 209; fasting for treatment of, 154–68; traditional treatments, 143
autolysis (self-digestion), 16
autonomic nervous system, 20
avocado, 137
Azulfidine, 143, 158

bacterial infections, 180
bananas, 83
barbiturates, 79, 80–81
barley, 166
barley mush, 55
beans, 40, 42, 187, 188. *See also* legumes
Beclovent, 158
beef, and lupus, 161
beef industry, USDA support for, 48
benign tumors, 176–77
beta-blockers, 118
beta carotene, 31, 37–38

beta cell function, 131, 135, 140
bilirubin, 207, 209
biofeedback, 81, 82
bioflavonoids, 31, 138
biologic concentration, 41
birth control pills, 81, 85, 159
bleeding, internal, 151
blindness, diabetes and, 127
blood–brain barrier, 78, 84
blood clotting, 9, 120
blood lipids, in diabetics, 127–28
blood pressure, 9, 15, 115–19, 201, 202–3, 222; high (*see* high blood pressure)
blood sugar levels, 127–28, 129. *See also* hypoglycemia
blood tests, 9, 206–10
body fat, 28–29, 52, 67–69, 130, 131, 133, 151, 186, 211
body temperature, 203, 218
Bogalusa Heart Study, 28–29
bone marrow destruction, 151
borage oil, 167, 171
bowel movements, 204, 219, 220, 223
brain function, 11, 32, 96–97, 104, 197–99
brain tumors, 82
bread, 40
breast cancer, 27, 34–36, 38, 41–42, 96
breast milk, 164–65
breast tumors, 176
broccoli, 40
buffalo hump, 151
BUN (blood urea nitrogen) test, 96, 207, 208
Burkitt, Dennis, 31–32
Burton, Alec, 175
bypass surgery, 102, 103–5, 111–12

caffeine, 42, 80–81, 84, 192, 211, 216. *See also* coffee
calcium, 39–41
calories, 16, 42–43, 69, 186–89

headaches, during fasting, 18–19, 73, 205
head injury, 82
"healing or fasting crisis," 223
health care, traditional, failure of, 1–2, 21–22, 57. *See also* physicians
health insurance, costs of, 48
"Healthy People 2000" program, 2
hearing loss, 151
heart attack, 24, 73–74, 102, 105, 115, 118, 119–20
heart disease, 25, 47, 52, 95, 101–26, 127–29. *See also* cardiovascular disease; coronary artery disease
Hegsted, Mark, 34
Helsinki health trial, 103
hemoglobin levels, 207
hemolytic anemia, 145–46
hemorrhoids, 30
heparin, 211
hepatitis, 112
herbs, 9, 10, 62, 85, 170
heroin, 80
herring, 83
heterocyclic amines, 41–42
hibernation, 13
high blood pressure, 1, 22, 101–2, 190; case histories, 116
high-protein, carbohydrate-restricted diets, 189–91
high-protein diet, 39–42, 84, 90, 95–98
Hippocrates, 16, 17, 55
Hippocratic Oath, 17, 22
Hodgkin's disease, 152
hormonal changes, during fasting, 197, 203
hormonal deficits, 89
hormone replacement, 201
hot baths, 170, 218
human body: cause-and-effect laws of disease and health in, 70–72; fasting as natural to, 11–14, 16–17, 191, 212, 213; self-healing

powers of, 3–4, 7–8, 13–14, 15–16, 23, 57, 58–62, 89, 169–70, 213; unsuited to high-protein diet, 33–34, 95–96, 148–49
hunger, 12, 18, 214, 215
hydration, 199, 202, 203, 204–5, 207–8, 222–23
hydrazines, 160
hyperactivity, 28
hypertension, 82, 112. *See* high blood pressure
hyperthyroidism, 113
hypoglycemia, 89–100, 135; case histories, 99–100
hypoglycemic pills, 135, 201
hypothyroidism, 192, 201
hysterectomy, 176

iatrogenic disease, 105
ice cream, 83
immune system, 14, 29–30, 32, 37, 68, 69–70, 144, 147–49, 155, 183
impotence, 101, 123–24
Imuran, 151
incoordination, 89
indole, 34
Indonesia, 153
infection, 155, 164
inflammation, 61, 146, 149–50, 182–84. *See also* rheumatoid arthritis
inflammatory bowel disease, 146, 164–68, 204
injury, body's reaction to, 182–84
insomnia, 151, 205
insulin, 90–91, 129–36, 141, 201
insulin-secreting tumors, 89
insulin surge, 91–92
interferon, 14, 68, 191
intermediate metabolites, 65–66
International Association of Professional Natural Hygienists, 195
intestinal bacteria, 45, 60, 148–49
intestinal spasm, 30

"cure" with traditional treatments, 102–5, 133–36, 143 (*see also* symptoms); responsibility to patients in treatment choices, 53–54, 112, 118, 212; supervision of fasting, 194–96, 199–201, 217
Physicians Committee for Responsible Medicine, 25
phytochemicals, 30, 37
Pima Indians, 132
pineapple, 220
plant-based diet, 18, 26, 29–31, 36, 40–41, 42–46, 52, 68, 73, 84, 95–97, 106–9, 125–26, 136–38, 148, 153–54
plaque, atherosclerotic, 15, 101–2, 113, 117, 119–20, 131, 133, 150, 209–10
Plaquenil, 151
platelet destruction, 151
Plato, 16
PMS, 28
poisoning, 19, 113
political fasts, 17
polymyalgia rheumatica, 191
porphyria, 200
potassium, 196, 208–9, 217, 220–21
potatoes, 167, 169, 189
poultry, 27
prednisone, 143, 150–51, 152, 158, 163, 167, 171
pregnancy, 159, 200
primrose oil, 167
processed foods, 26, 28, 29, 31–32, 52, 68
proctitis, 62, 166
prostate cancer, 27, 36
prostatitis, 61
protein, 26, 68, 95–98, 147–50, 161; animal vs. plant, 40–41, 95–96, 97, 148, 160; RDA, 39–40; sources of, 40–41; toxins in metabolism of, 96–97. *See also* animal-based diet; high-protein diet

protein-modified fasts, 191
protein sparing, 9, 12, 198, 211, 215
proteolytic bacteria, 34
psoralens, 160
psoriasis, 1, 20, 146, 151, 153, 159, 209
psoriatic arthritis, 153, 159
psychological disorders, 19
psychosis, 151
puberty, early, and cancer, 27, 36, 96
pulse pressure, 203
purines, 206, 207
pyridoxine, 33
Pythagoras, 16

rapid heart beat, 89
rashes, 60, 62, 73, 135, 151, 181, 223
Ray, Earl, 132
reactive (functional) hypoglycemia, 89, 90–100
Recommended Dietary Allowance (RDA), 31, 39–40, 44
red meat, 41, 107
refined foods, 28, 31–32, 42
relaxation, progressive, 81
religious fasts, 17
renal function, 89, 95, 102
repair, body's natural power to, 182–84, 218
respiratory infections, 113
restenosis, 105
retinal damage, 151
rheumatic fever, 113
rheumatoid arthritis, 22, 95, 143, 146, 149, 152–58; case histories, 157–58, 171
rhinitis, 144
rhinorrhea, 223
rice, 167
Rockefeller Institute for Medical Research (New York), 139
rosacea, 176
rutin, 138
rye, 166, 167

salad, 137
salicylates, 150
salted foods, 83
schizophrenia, 151
secretory IgA, 165
seeds, 42, 87
Seldane, 158
selenium, 37
self-hypnosis, 81
senile dementia, 101
septic meningitis, 150
serotonin, 119
serum bicarbonate, 203
serum immunoglobulin levels, 70
serums, 170
Seventh-Day Adventists, 74–75
sexual dysfunction, 101, 119, 123–24
shaking, 89
Shelton, Herbert, 17, 56–57, 206–7, 217
Shelton's Health School, 5, 56–57
sinusitis, 20, 83, 87, 178–82
sinus rhythm, 204
Sjögren's syndrome, 144
skatole, 34
skin, 61. See also rashes
skin testing response, 70
sleep, 72, 218
Socrates, 16
sodium, 43, 121–22, 208
soft drinks, 42, 80, 85
soy beans, 160
soy oil, 29
spinach, 160, 161
starvation, 12–13, 70, 196–97, 204, 210
steamed/stewed vegetables, 167, 168, 202, 220
steroids, 150–51, 158, 159, 162, 163, 183, 200–201
stomach cancer, 38
stomach lining, irritation of, 150
stretching exercises, 218
stroke, 24, 102, 105, 115, 120
sucrose, 166
sugar industry, 50

sugars, 166
suicide, 151
sulfamethazine, 41
sunbathing, 203, 218
superoxide dismutase complex, 138
suppressor T cells, 162
surgery, 1, 21, 71, 119. See also bypass surgery
sweating, 89
sweeteners, 28, 42, 83
sweets, 26
swelling, 118, 150, 225
symptoms, suppressing with medication vs. curing, 13–14, 21, 61, 71, 103, 182–84
systemic lupus erythematosus (SLE), 1, 95, 146, 153, 157, 159–64; case histories, 162–64

T cell activity, 70
tea, 8, 85, 167
tension headaches, 93
theophylline, 211
thrombophlebitis, 121
thrombus, 119–20
thyroid tumors, 41
Tilden, John, 56
tinnitis, 150, 191
Tohono O'odham Indians, 132
tomatoes, 169
tongue, coated, 73, 222
toxicosis, 59, 62–63, 170
toxins, 8, 59–60, 76, 77–81, 96–97
tranquilizers, 201
transdermal clonidine patch, 201
triglycerides, 38, 127–28, 210
tuberculosis, 82, 151
tumors, 69
Twain, Mark, 17

ulcerative colitis, 1, 146, 164–68
ulcers, 112, 150
undereating, 69–70
urea, 92, 96, 97
uric acid, 34, 97, 206–7
urinalyses, 206